The Gentle Path

to
Definitive Weight Loss

Rachel Norwood

To my Mother,
Martha Brodie Hurlstone
9th October 1942 – 17th October 2007,
With Love...

Acknowledgements:

There are a number of people who I am very grateful to for their help and encouragement in getting this book to see the light of day. The journey over this last year writing this book has been adventurous and enlightening; my eternal Thanks and Love go out to the following people:

Tammy Furey, *Three Principles Practitioner, Specialist in Parenting, for her tireless, gentle and loving contribution to the editing of this book http://3principlesparenting.wordpress.com/*

Reverend Malcolm Clarke *for his support and enthusiasm and his help in the editing process*

Katri Manninen, *Certified Transformative Supercoach and Three Principles Practitioner, for her encouragement and love in allowing me to find the space for inspiration to begin the writing process http://katrimanninen.net/in-english/*

Michael Neill, *Supercoach and wonderful teacher of the inside out understanding of the human experience, without whose teaching I would not have been able to clearly put into words many of the psychological clicks that came about within my own experience all those years ago, enabling me to share them with you in this book http://www.supercoach.com/*

*To **all my Clients** who have been a true source of inspiration in the work that I carry out*

*To my children, **Alistair and Colleen**, for their excitement and enthusiasm... "Mummy's written a book!"*

Table of Contents:

Introduction

Once upon a time...

Once upon a time, in a not so far away land, a beautiful baby girl was born. She was a normal, chubby little thing with porcelain skin and soft dark curls. Her mother had type I diabetes and though she was a perfectly healthy baby, the wicked Wizard Obesity had put an enchantment on her and he was always watching, ready to pounce and ensnare her.

During her childhood, she went through phases of putting on weight and then losing it again but as she grew older, the enchantment of the wicked Wizard became stronger and stronger, making her put on more and more weight each time and losing less and less, until one day she became so overweight that even walking was difficult.

She then visited all the witch doctors in the land in search of a remedy but nothing worked, and as time went on she became heavier and heavier and more and more tired and desperate to be relieved of the evil curse.

She read all the spell books that she could find on how to relieve the curse of the wicked Wizard Obesity. She tried many magic potions and powders to free herself of her plague, but all to no avail.

One day, after much searching in old places of learning for secret, hidden books written by Wizards of a Higher Order, and wandering through the wide, vast wilderness in the land of Inter Net, the good fairy Common Sense visited her. The young woman, with the help of the good fairy Common Sense, put together a plan of action. By using these new enchantments they worked together until, in a very short space of time, she had finally alleviated the evil spell for ever and the wicked Wizard Obesity was no more...

*And they all lived **healthily** ever after!*

Dear Reader,

Someone told me once that the introduction to a book should be written at the end of the writing process. Not listening to that advice, I had initially written an introduction explaining in bland terms who I am and what I do, etc.

As I was writing the book, it became more and more apparent that my original introduction didn't fit in with what this book is about. You see, this book isn't about me; it's about you.

Every single word held within these pages was written directly from my heart. I realized, somewhere between having the idea of writing this book and its subsequent completion, I was writing with a sense of purpose. Everything that happened in my life had led me to this point of wanting to write this book. I wanted to share my experience in the hope of helping others who may be experiencing what I went through myself.

You are probably asking yourself, and I certainly hope you are, why this book is different from any other diet book out there on the market?

Well, a lot of books dictate what you should and shouldn't eat, whilst carrying threats of failure if you do not follow to the letter everything that is written within. This book is different: there are no meal plans with precise menus to follow. I am not going to lecture you or try to make you feel inferior. I don't believe that you need to feel bad about yourself in order to do something about your weight problem. I am convinced that you already know what to do; my objective is just to give you a very gentle nudge to get you onto that *Gentle Path to Definitive Weight Loss*.

This book is not about short-term dieting. It is about a lifelong awareness of our eating habits so that we can enjoy what we eat and gain enormous health and energy.

I wasn't always overweight, as you will read, but I have always had a tendency to put on weight easily and, as for many people, have gone through the torment of fighting to lose that weight. Heavily obese for a period of five to ten years, one day something clicked into place. I will be sharing in this book how that click came about.

Using the knowledge that I had gained over so many years of fighting against being overweight, I put into place my own eating principles. They are not based on a doctor's prescription or a diet. I have drawn from the best of what I learned and have created my own way of doing things.

The surprising part is, the measures that I put into place have little or nothing to do with what we are habitually told to do in order to lose weight. I discovered that many of the different methods, whether recommended or not, are in fact counterproductive.

This book is also different for the very simple fact that I have been there, exactly where you might be right now. Very simply, I completely identify with what you may be going through. I know what it feels like, how upsetting and frustrating it is, how hurtful the looks of others and the unpleasant comments and even insults, are.

* I've been through the embarrassment of enrolling at the local gym in an effort to better myself. Other members, and even some instructors, mocked me and didn't recognise the health I was aspiring to regain.

* I've been in the medical office of the pretty, thin nutritionist who condescendingly told me that I was fat because I simply ate too much. Her solution was to more or less stop eating.

* I've been to that hellish place looking desperately for a rapid solution to the weight problem that was hurting me both physically and psychologically, so desperate that I would at times undertake actions that were detrimental to both my health and to what I was hoping to achieve.

* I've been to that dinner party where relatives and friends have made fun of me at the moment of serving the meal with remarks such as "no point giving her too much, she can use her reserves!" and then seeing myself presented with a much smaller portion than everybody else.

Above all, this book is different because I want you to look on it as a conversation between you and me. I want you to always be aware of your own thinking because, ultimately, I'm not going to tell you what to do. My goal is to bring you to a place where you know exactly what YOU want to do and you then go and do what is right for you. If you disagree with me then good, as long as you are listening to your own intuition and inner voice of wisdom, then you can be fully confident that you are on the right path.

I will be sharing many of the preconceived ideas around dieting and weight loss; my goal is to help you sweep those ideas away, giving you space to form your own ideas and opinions. When you are comfortably in that place in you where you're doing what feels right for you, then that is what is going to work the best and help you get the results that you're aspiring to achieve.

I See the Light in You,
Rachel

My Story

"There is no sincerer love than the love of food"
George Bernard Shaw

I've always had a weight problem, a tendency to put on weight easily. At the same time I have a great love and passion for food. I love the taste of delicious food; I love the smell of food cooking, when the aromas fill the house. I love sitting down to a nice tasty meal... Who doesn't? This short autobiography is about how I came to lose weight while still appreciating and loving the food that I eat.

Looking back on photographs, it is clear I was overweight around the age of three. At the time I was staying with my grandparents who were very kind, especially my Gran who sang and smiled. She also made lots of lovely food.

I remember soft-boiled eggs in the morning with buttered "soldiers", watching the egg timer hungrily until the minutes were up. I remember bangers and mash (sausages and mashed potatoes, for those of you who are unfamiliar with the more exquisite British culinary terms). I remember baked beans on toast and scrambled eggs. I remember thick cut homemade chips with tomato ketchup. I remember oranges with sugar sprinkled over the top, the sugar crystallising with the juice from the fruit and turning crunchy. I remember thick homemade Scotch broth with buttered bread and "boats". I remember lots of sweeties!
What I don't remember is putting on weight but I did.

By the age of four I had come back to a normal weight for a little girl. Back home my mother with her dieting knowledge through dealing with type I diabetes, put me on a regimen with more whole foods, vegetables, leaner meat, and the sweeties were rationed out. We also had lots of walks through the Scottish countryside, plenty of fresh air and outdoor activities.

When I was six my Gran died of cancer and a very short time afterwards, it felt like only a matter of weeks, our family moved from Scotland to the Midlands, England. I found myself in a totally new environment with new people, new friends and a new school, whilst overcoming a major loss in our family.

We were living on an army camp. The army people living there were honest and moral but not very rich, often with several small mouths to feed. At that time, in the seventies, the government provided free school meals and, for some families, such as the army, the free school dinner meant that their children got the only decent meal that they would have in the day.
To ensure that the children received enough food to fill them up, we were allowed second and even third helpings. The meals consisted of meat or fish with starch foods, potatoes, rice and pasta. The sauces were systematically thickened with flour. Occasionally vegetables found their way into the meals. We were also served a ration of milk at break time in the morning. I also had a full dinner when I got home.

And so, once again, I started gaining weight and again my mother intervened. The school dinners were stopped and I was given a packed lunch, usually a wholemeal bread sandwich with a piece of fruit as dessert; once a week a biscuit or a packet of crisps would find their way into my sandwich box. The sandwich nearly always contained some kind of vegetable – tomato, salad and onion. And again, the weight came off.

As any normal healthy child, I was very active – cycling, running, playing with my friends, climbing trees. We were also very lucky to be living right in the middle of the countryside, which allowed for plenty of fresh air.

I maintained, for many years, what would be considered a normal weight. I wasn't always as thin as some of my friends but I was a normal weight.

The next time I put on weight was when I had just got into my twenties. In my first year at university, I was perfectly normal but my eating habits perhaps left a little to be desired; although at that time I also adopted a vegetarian style diet so was eating more vegetables – mostly soup! My friends who have known me since those university years can confirm what a gourmet cook I was! I would invite them round for dinner and regularly serve them up helpings of soup and mushed-up gunge! Have you ever seen the first of the Bridget Jones films? Do you remember the classic birthday dinner that she cooked for her friends? You get the picture! Happily I have learned since how to cook properly and make nicer food that not only tastes good but looks good too!

At that same time, I had got into the habit of drinking the light version of a famous grape juice drink and I was drinking at least three or four of those little cartons every day.
Then I found myself in a serious relationship. My fiancé, however, was not vegetarian and didn't believe in whole foods. I went back to a meat-based diet and started eating, on a daily basis, ham or cheese and pickle sandwiches, richer foods, starch at every mealtime, pizzas, hamburgers, chips, etc, etc.

I literally ballooned up in a matter of weeks. The sudden change in the diet had an abrupt and drastic effect on my body. Within a few short weeks I had to get myself a new wardrobe as none of my clothes fitted!
This was the heaviest I had ever been in my life, a whopping 63kg for my 5'1"!
I tried, for the first time in my life, to diet on my own. I put myself on a starvation diet, rationing out all the

food, with no more than one slice of bread a day and carefully weighing out every bit of food that was going to be eaten.

Did I lose weight? Nope!

Was I hungry? Extremely!

Was I tired and grumpy? Absolutely!

Was it a pleasant experience? Definitely not!

In a bid to fight off the hunger pangs I bought myself appetite suppressants, the result of that was that I felt nauseous, my stomach hurt and I still felt hungry!

I stayed at that weight for two or three years until I came to France.

It was when I came to France that I started reading many books on how to lose weight and on nutrition in general. This was the time before the internet - when books and journals were the main resources for learning – does anyone remember that?! I have, in fact, been researching the subject of nutrition for nigh on twenty years.

I got hooked on the Montignac method and actually lost the weight. I got down to a lovely 48kg, though my mother thought I was too thin; but then Mothers always worry that their children aren't eating enough!

But then I hit a roadblock, I gained about 6kg, which is nothing dramatic and I was still well within what is considered to be normal but no matter how hard I tried, I couldn't get back down to the weight that I felt I should be. It was really frustrating!

Again followed a long period where I remained at a normal weight... until 2002-2003 when disaster struck.

I found myself at a heady 77kg with little idea how that came about. Later I realised, and throughout this book you will discover why that happened and how I managed to get the weight off and keep it off since.

In 2004, I fell pregnant with my first child and I put on 10kg, which is a perfectly normal weight gain for a pregnancy. Once my son was born however, I stayed at that weight, which was around 83kg to 84kg.

In 2006, I fell pregnant with my second child. Again a weight gain of around 10kg and again the weight didn't come off. In fact, once my daughter was born, I gained even more weight and reached a shocking 93kg.

It was a nightmare! How ugly and bizarre I felt looking at myself in the mirror and not recognizing myself! I was in pain, both psychologically and physically. I had trouble walking and balancing myself. I got out of breath bending down to do up my shoes. I needed up to fifteen minutes in the morning to get out of bed and straighten up, that's how painful my back was. I had excruciating pains in my ankles and knees that would come on very suddenly. The simplest movements were exhausting and it was a struggle to get in and out of the car. It was uncomfortable, painful and unpleasant!

I tried everything – every diet that was on the market. I went to see doctors, nutritionists and specialists. None of it worked. All of the diets that I was prescribed, or that I self-prescribed, were really difficult to put in place and maintain. The only result was my own disappointment and desperation.

And then, very suddenly, something happened. Something clicked into place. Everything I had been reading about nutrition and dieting suddenly started to make sense to me. The big advantage was that the internet was up and running, giving me access to a fountain of knowledge, if you knew where to look and the right key words to search with. I discovered information about certain foods that would make your hair stand on end, shocking information that is never divulged to us.

And so with my newfound common sense I worked out my own plan, based on the knowledge that I had gained and I ate! I ate myself back into health. I didn't worry about amounts, and am definitely not going to suggest to you that you reduce your food intake in any way, but I became very naturally *mindful* of how and what I was eating.

I let go and I stopped fighting. I decided that I was not going to lose weight but that I would at least take care of myself on the inside. I stopped beating myself up every time I looked in the mirror and I stopped weighing myself. I basically started accepting myself for who I was at that time, I decided to beautify myself from the inside out, and everyone knows beauty comes from the inside...

I was no longer in pain psychologically and, through taking care of my inner self, physically and emotionally, the weight started dropping...   miraculously and effortlessly.

I changed my eating habits around May to June 2008. During the course of the summer holidays I lost around 20kg. People, who hadn't seen me since the holidays, would walk past me, as they simply didn't recognize me. And that was a nice feeling I have to admit!

Over the next five to six months I dropped another 25kg making a total weight loss of around 45kg – I again had to go out and get myself a new wardrobe, but this time it was a real pleasure to do so!

The eating habits that I put in place at that time, and that I continue to use as a principle for my every day eating, are very simple. I want you to know why they work so that you can find the ideal way of eating for yourself but most of all I want to get over to you the psychological change in the mindset that allowed all of that to so easily and effortlessly click into place.

I could have just written a leaflet with how I eat on a daily basis and presented that, but it would serve no purpose to you. What we must do, is shine the light on why we put on weight, why it is so difficult to lose weight, emotionally and physically, through all the dieting techniques that are out there and how you can lose the weight and get back to your health…. definitively!

A lot of what is written here is just basic common sense and some of this you may already know, but it's good to have a reminder and a fair bit of support for your own ideas.

I hope you will enjoy reading this book and that you will get a lot out of it. Knowledge is power, especially when it comes to eating habits and losing weight.

Part 1

Homo Sapiens to Homo Fatiens

Why "Traditional" Dieting Doesn't Work

"Let food be your medicine and medicine be your food"
"Wherever the art of Medicine is loved, there is also a love of Humanity"
Hippocrates

We live in an amazing time! We have so much technology and information to hand; means of communicating that people, just one hundred years ago, could never even have dreamt of. With a little effort we are assured of at least getting by with a fairly decent life (at least in the Western world!) We have developed means of transportation that allow us to transport goods and experience them from the four corners of the globe. We can also travel to these places to absorb different and unique cultures.

We have developed means of obtaining food that no longer involve hunting or lengthy processes of preparation. We can freely go to restaurants and eat to our heart's content. We have machines to take care of the housework, thus giving us, apparently, more time to concentrate on our families, our professional activities and our leisure time.

We have hypermarkets, drive-ins, and delivery services. We have "Feast-on-Call" literally at our fingertips!

With the very rapid development of the Western world, we have also developed means of mass production, but through that we are destroying the very environment that supports us for life. We are transforming everything, even to the food that we eat – refining, processing, genetically modifying, spraying pesticides, fungicides, chemical fertilizers, weed killers...

We have created a society where the food that we eat has little or nothing to do with its original form and taste. From the moment a vegetable is planted as a seed to the moment that it reaches our table, it has gone through so many different processes, that it can end up being devoid of its original nutrients, vitamins and minerals. Farm animals are fed genetically modified foods and are pumped full of antibiotics and growth hormones. All of those elements finish up, invisibly and inevitably, on our plates.

We are using our industrial and technological knowledge neither to nurture nor honour this beautiful Earth that we are so lucky to inhabit. Rather we are creating a society of greed and dependence, based on financial gain.

And it is becoming less and less possible to obtain simple, natural food.

When you walk through a supermarket, the shelves are stacked high with processed, refined, transformed foods. Aisles that stock the simple, natural foods are few and far between, and less and less easy to find.

With all of this mass production, you would think that nobody should go hungry. But we do!

Human beings have, since the beginning of our time, always eaten the foods that were readily available. And Nature is marvellous! Every food available on this planet is complete from a nutritional point of view, as long as you eat the whole thing!

The problem, the major problem, with our society today, is that the readily available foods are no longer the ones that we pick from trees, lift from the ground, fish and hunt. They are the ones that we are buying in the supermarkets, the hypermarkets, the fast-food restaurants.

When you walk through a supermarket, the shelves are packed to the brim with these nutritional by-products. They have been so processed and refined that there is nothing left, most of the time, not even the taste. And so that they do, indeed, taste of something, we add sugars, flavourings, salts, sodium glutamate, chemical products. This is no longer food, but this is, unfortunately, what is readily available.

Our bodies are wonderful organisms but they need a certain amount of nutriments, vitamins and minerals every day in order to maintain our health and energy, that's common knowledge. But, in order to obtain the amount of nutriments, vitamins and minerals necessary for our vital functions we have no choice but to consume huge amounts of these mass-produced foods.

Since the coming of man, our body has been programmed to seek out the food that meets our nutritional requirements and these "programs" have been tried and proven throughout time. One of the programs running in our body is our capacity to desire foods that contain the nutriments that we may be lacking; this is our basic intuition.

Easily recognizable, especially among pregnant women throughout the world, this basic instinct is also known as cravings. When the baby that is growing inside the womb requires a particular nutriment to enable its growth, the mother gets a craving for the food that contains the most of it. I remember when I was carrying my son, my cravings were so strong that I could eat a kilo of green olives a day!

But this doesn't only concern pregnant women. If your body is claiming vitamin C, for example, it's going to look for foods containing vitamin C, very naturally.
The problem is, and this seems very logical, that if the vitamin C in the mass-produced food item that you are eating is practically non-existent, your body, claiming that vitamin, is going to require you to eat or drink far more of that particular food or beverage in order to

cover the vital needs.

This brings us to the next problem, the consumption of huge amounts of these industrially-produced, transformed, non-natural foods that often contain additives, sugars and chemical preservatives that wreak havoc on our bodies' internal systems and vital organs.
The most obvious and apparent sign of this havoc is putting on weight to the point of being so obese that, for some, we end up needing a walking aid or a wheelchair to get around.
And that's without mentioning all of the other obesity related illnesses and diseases. Yet, despite the huge quantities of food and the ever-growing weight/obesity problem we are still undernourished.

What is the difference between a starving child in Africa and an obese child in the Western world?

To my mind, there is very little difference. The starving child is suffering from severe malnutrition and will die if nothing is done. The obese child is also suffering from severe malnutrition, but on a completely different level. Death may not be an immediate consequence; this obese child will have the pleasure of going through some pretty nasty chronic illnesses as he/she grows up. If nothing is done, this child will also die, maybe not in his/her younger years but their life span will be vastly reduced.

Basically, we are overeating this kind of food to the point of being morbidly obese... but we are still starving!

Now, I know what you're probably thinking! "Wait a minute, she said that this didn't have anything to do with portion control or weighing food, etc. Now she's going to tell us to eat less!"

Well, not exactly. First of all, I'm not here to tell you what to do. My goal is to give you the information so that you can make your own choices.
But I am here to tell you this "Don't eat less! Eat better!"

So let's take a look at that...

The Diet Market

"Believe nothing, no matter where you read it or who has said it, not even if I have said it, unless it agrees with your own reason and your own common sense"
Buddha

Obesity, in a certain sense, has always existed. We can look back into history and find rare cases. We see it amongst the Ancient Egyptians, we find it within the Roman Empire, we find it in most every society that has achieved a state of opulence.
But since the beginning of the 20th century, the growing problem of obesity had never been at such a high level, nor so widespread as it is today, reaching the gargantuan proportions that we see around us every day, as much in the amount of people suffering from the affliction as to the size of the people themselves.
With this very sudden appearance of widespread obesity has come the flourishing of a new market – the diet market.

This diet market is made up of researchers, doctors, nutritionist, scientists, government officials, food lobbyists, the big food conglomerates, pharmaceutical companies, etc. Some are sincerely there to try and find a solution to the problem but there are others who, very simply, do not want a solution; while we get more and more fat, so do their wallets!

Of course, the problem is searching out the right information, knowing where to look and who to believe. Governments regularly issue public health recommendations telling us how and what we should be eating but few of these papers are neutral. The big food companies who are either partly or wholly responsible for the obesity problem finance many of these studies; they are the starting point of the problem – they are the ones producing the foods. And they need us to keep eating their food otherwise they would purely and simply go out of business – at least, that's what they believe and fear.

The latest initiative to date was the "five-a-day" rule (for those not in the EU, the rule is to eat five fresh fruit and vegetables per day). We are led to believe that if we have a continuing weight or obesity problem, it is our own fault because we're not following whatever recommendations happen to be in vogue.

On the other hand, who can blame us? A walk through the supermarket, there are so many tempting refined, processed, easy-to-cook, easy-to-eat products – how do we even know where to start looking for the five-a-day?

And then, when you think about it, did ancient man worry about eating five-a-day? Did the tribe leaders get together one day and decide that all those who did not eat five-a-day should have a hole put in their heads? No, ancient man just ate what was there, as do we today…. largely to our detriment.

Previously, there was the "balanced-meal" rule. A meal should contain protein, vegetable and starch, in certain proportions, and many people still think that is true today.

However, until the 1700s, man did not mix carbohydrate and fat on the same plate.

Man would eat carbohydrate only during times of famine when there was nothing else available. Another important point to bear in mind is that carbohydrate, particularly in the form that it is eaten today, exists nowhere in Nature.

"What about bread?" Well, bread has been around for a really long time, since man discovered the art of agriculture. Ancient bread, however, has little in common with the refined, white, sugared, vinegary,

salted by-product that we buy in plastic packaging today.
Bread was also used as a means of transporting a meal – this was the time before cling-film and salad bags! The bread itself was not necessarily eaten but instead served to protect the food that was held within.

The wheat flour that we use today for our bread is not the original, prehistoric wheat. Around ten thousand years ago, which is very recent in our history, the Ancient Egyptians found a way of modifying the wheat in order to make bread that was more supple and softer, and this "new" wheat became the wheat that we know today – heavily loaded with gluten. Add to that the refining processes, all the preservatives and chemicals and bread is no longer a healthy product. Yet, that is not what we are told.

There is so much <u>mis</u>information out there that we get to the stage where we have no idea what to do or how to eat.

One of the challenges that we face is accepting to let go of all our preconceived ideas. We are, in all honesty, brainwashed into thinking that certain foods are healthy. Turn on the TV and you have the latest "pro-biotic" milk product, which is logically more expensive because it has that extra-something. The publicity informs us that without it we won't get through the winter and that we absolutely need it to boost our immune system.
The trouble is, of course, that once these products have been pasteurised, most often ultra heat treated, processed, packaged and transported to the end of the food chain, the "pro-biotic" elements are not any higher than any other ordinary yoghurt, if existent at all. Not to mention the addition of sugar and flavouring, as in their natural state these mini-yoghurt drinks taste so bad that they would make you, at best, spit them out.

A person I was working with got very upset one day at the idea of not having a dessert at the end of a meal. To her knowledge, a dessert was something that is necessary, even from a health point of view. She believed that the dessert, rich in sugar, would use up the excess insulin in the body. Again, this is a misleading preconception.

So how do we nudge these preconceived ideas?
I encourage you to question everything that you hear, particularly if there is a big marketing campaign behind it. I believe in every single person's capacity to make intelligent, informed and wise decisions. This isn't "rocket science" though we are often led to believe so. Understanding how the human body works and becoming aware of your own intuition is essential. You have that capacity. Every single person on Earth has that innate ability to use intuition and wisdom.

The Chinese say that our food is our first medicine. Now I'm not ruling out modern medicine, and I am aware that in many cases modern medicine is indispensable. I am definitely not telling you to very suddenly stop taking medication that you may have been prescribed, only a doctor can advise you in that regard, for that could be a terrible mistake for your health and perhaps even your life.
However, the problem with modern medicine is that we tend to treat the symptoms without finding the source.
You could see it like this: if a stream is flowing with toxic substances from the source, you can clean up the area where you live that is poisoned, but if you don't clear it up at the source then no matter how much you attempt to purify your part of the stream, the toxicity is going to keep coming back.

So back to the diet market! And just to give you one of those little nudges to help you question:
With all the diets, papers, advice and information

available, it's unbelievable that the obesity problem is actually getting worse instead of better.

If you're like me and have tried out many different kinds of diets and ended up putting on weight instead of losing it, we have to ask "WHY?"

These diets are great! They all have enticing names, often incorporating the name of the "doctor" or "scientist" who has written the latest book that is loaded with 'miracles.' They are almost always accompanied by subliminal promises – "Do this diet and you will become perfect: look like Julia Roberts/George Clooney: get lots of hot dates with Julia Roberts/George Clooney!" (I have a personal preference for a hot date with Tom Hanks, but only because he looks a little like my husband!)

These diets, more often than not, make promises that appeal to our need for love, whether in our personal relationships or acceptance in society. They touch our fear of being rejected and play on our instinct for survival.

I've yet to see an advertisement with someone overweight, sexily putting the spoon of "light dessert" into his or her mouth. We are plagued by images of happy families, laughing together, all enjoying the latest "healthy" or not so healthy product. We are, if we're honest, psychologically manipulated into believing that we have to eat a certain way, be and live a certain way and have certain things in order to be happy and successful. But I like to make up my own mind and I encourage you to do the same (and this includes anything that you read in this book).

My motto is: ***do what works best for you!***

Listening and taking all of this marketing mumbo-jumbo on board, led me to a very long period of confusion and frustration. I didn't know what the heck to eat and

EVERY mouthful was a GUILTY mouthful. Have you ever been there? Perhaps that is how you are feeling right now?

I couldn't help thinking to myself, "if all of these products are so healthy, why am I not losing weight? Why am I not healthier? Why isn't everybody thin and healthy?"

Here are a few answers to those questions...

The Low-Calorie Con

Restrictive, frustrating and unsatisfying - and I have done a lot of those diets in my time!

They always start out being fabulous and fun... for the first half day! The careful weighing out of food, making sure to not be even a milligram over the prescribed amount so as not to go above the daily allowance of calorie intake is quite a pleasure – you are happy because you feel that you are doing something nice for yourself and, *"ta-da!"* From this moment on you are going to take care, look good, feel like a sexy million dollars, be perfectly healthy AND get that hot date!

But, here's the thing that got me: I would find myself looking at a really nice meal on my plate... but there just was not enough of it! So I would chew it very slowly to make it last just that little bit longer, I mean they tell us we should chew our food slowly and carefully, don't they? All to no avail, I was still hungry at the end of the meal!

Can you think of anything worse than leaving the table still hungry? Do animals in nature do that? D'ya think ancient man did that? Well, they do, and they did, but only if there isn't/wasn't enough food!

To my mind, this is along the same lines as those who say that you MUST stop eating just before you get to the stage of satiety. How frustrating! You have something really nice on your plate and though you still feel hungry and your appetite is still there, you have to use a force that Superman would be proud of to push the plate away! Hands up if you find that satisfying? Some cultures would consider this behaviour to be absurd and even bad manners!

By all means, if you really have had enough, then obviously stop, the idea is not to make yourself feel sick, but please: eat enough.

There is much debate among the medical, health, nutrition, psychology and spiritual worlds on the subject of overeating. And everyone has his or her own opinion. Studies on leptin, the hunger regulating hormone, and its lack of production in severely obese mice that have a tendency to overeating, have led many to conclude that the solution is to eat less, though goodness only knows how they have come to that conclusion. These conclusions come in support of low-calorie dieting, which has been proven to be inefficient long-term.

Here is why under eating, which is the ultimate outcome of low-calorie dieting, does not work.

The body is a far more complex organism than we could even hope to fathom out. The proof of that is the quantity of studies that continue to be carried out on the human body. We may have walked on the moon but we still don't know all there is to know about the intricate workings of our own organism. Despite this obvious state of complexity and confusion, numerous scientists, doctors and government officials tell us what we should be eating in very simplistic terms.

So here's the simplistic low-calorie THEORY, which, you may be interested to know, was disproved by the same scientists that brought it out in the first place. The human body needs such and such an amount of calories; eat more than you need and you put on weight; eat less than you need you will lose weight; eat just the right amount and you will remain stable. Those simplistic statements raise some interesting questions.

The first question that ever came to my mind with regards to this, after having unsuccessfully tried many of these diets, was the following:

Given that I need and am eating, let's say, 2000 calories a day to maintain normal body function, it follows that I should reduce my intake to, let's say, 1500 calories a day in order to lose weight. Conversely, we're told that we SHOULD be eating 2000 calories a day. So at some point, in order to maintain normal body function, we're going to have to increase the amount of calories to be within the norm. Surely this will make us put on weight again, according to the theory? When you look at it from a very logical point of view, the theory actually makes no sense.

The second question that occurred to me was that we are told women actually need more nutrients than men, mostly to do with maintenance of our bodies for reproduction, and yet, most diet advertising is targeted at women. I am aware that men are more and more concerned with dieting and appearance, but it is still largely female based targeting. So, if women need more nutrients than men in order to survive and be healthy, why are we then subjecting ourselves to these low-calorie, portion-controlled diets where we are under nourishing ourselves in order to lose weight? It's completely contradictory.

The miracle of the human body is so complex and so beautifully designed and is entirely programmed for survival; here's really what happens when we go on a low-calorie diet: Our bodies very simply adapt to the new calorie intake and, where at the outset we saw a certain loss of weight, we now see it stabilizing. If you're like I was, the next step is to beat ourselves up – "We must be doing something wrong! We've not been careful enough!" And so then what do we do? We lower the calorie intake even more. The same thing then happens: we lose a bit and then we stabilize. Darn!

At this point we do one of two things – EITHER we give

up, thinking "we're totally unsuccessful, big fat slobs and rubbish at everything we do!" OR we lower the calorie intake even more; after all we are determined to beat this! Big mistake! Now your brain thinks there's a famine on so, not only will you not be losing any more weight, your body, not knowing how long the famine period will last, will actually start stocking energy in the form of fat cells in order to survive through the period until normal menus are restored. Just like a squirrel storing nuts to survive the winter period when there is little or no food, or like a bear fattening itself up in order to get through the period of hibernation.

And here's my theory on the leptin, an ordinary person's opinion based on simple logic. I believe that the leptin kicks in without any problem when the needs in nutrients are covered – it seems kind of commonsensical, doesn't it?
When you think of how much all of these mass-produced, processed, packaged and transported foods lack nutritional value, it's not surprising, to me in any case, that the leptin won't kick in. And even less surprising, to my mind, are the people who eat tonnes of these processed foods; they're not greedy, they're simply trying to cover their bodies' needs in necessary vitamins and minerals. The leptin is not kicking in because we are actually undernourished, despite the mass production and the super-availability of food.

I remember when I was still in high school we had music lessons in Paisley town on Saturday mornings. We would all meet up at lunchtime in the local fast food joint. One of my friends, a lovely young man, would have one of the menus and, complaining that he still felt hungry, would systematically go back and have a second portion. (Again, to be very clear, I'm not against second portions, this is about the quality not the quantity of the food that we eat) At the time, I thought, "wow, he's got a big appetite!" but now I realize he was just looking to be nourished with food that was practically, if not completely, empty of anything good. Another example of that is one of my relatives who I have seen eating five big macs in a row, again not because he's a glutton and doesn't know how to control himself but because he was also looking for nourishment.

Here's what I find when I eat that kind of food, which I do very occasionally; my stomach feels full but I don't feel that I've got anything from the meal and very rapidly, within two hours of eating in one of those places, I'm physically hungry again.

Slimfast & Co.

Meal substitutes?! That term, in itself, should carry a siren warning! The accompanying advertisement pitch usually goes along the lines of "a healthy substitute for a meal".

If you were to say that to your Granny, she'd burst out laughing!

But the psychological implications are terrible because the underlying meaning is that a normal meal made up of meat, fish, eggs, vegetables, etc is not as healthy as some powdered junk diluted in water! In order to dupe us, they are employing very clever advertising techniques and strategies that destabilize our own wisdom and common sense.

Often they employ celebrities to carry their campaigns through the media. The celebrity will explain how efficient the product is and how much weight they've lost using it; we're left believing, "well, if the celebrity does it, then surely it must be okay!" I would like to imagine that the celebrities who are paid to advertise such trash do so in all innocence. I also hope that they've never really tried these products themselves.

The advertising goes on to tell us that the substitute covers, in the particular case of one popular substitute meal drink, 1/3 of the "guideline daily amount" in vitamins and minerals per portion. That's quite handy as you're supposed to have 3 of these substitutes a day. BUT, they give the whole game away when they finish by saying 3 substitute meals, 2 *insert company name here* snacks, plus 1 **sensible meal**. So, why not just have sensible meals throughout the day and forget about the substitutes? I mean, seriously!

Even more deceiving is when you look at the list of ingredients, which according to the company's advertising are healthy ingredients that are going to help you lose weight. For the sake of argument, I did a little research and would like to present you with a small comparison.

Here is the list of ingredients for a famous meal substitute chocolate drink:

> *Skimmed Milk (78%), Water, Milk Proteins, Cocoa Powder (1.2%), Vegetable Oil, Sugar, Stabilisers (Cellulose, Cellulose Gum, Dipotassium Phosphate, Carrageenan), Thickener (Gum Arabic), Maltodextrin, Emulsifiers (Mono- and Diglycerides of Fatty Acids), Vitamins and Minerals*, Sweeteners (Sucralose, Acesulfame-K), Flavourings, Antioxidant (Ascorbic Acid),*
> **Vitamins and Minerals: Potassium Chloride, Sodium Carbonate, Magnesium Hydroxide, Vitamin C, Sodium Chloride, Zinc Gluconate, Vitamin E, Ferric Pyrophosphate, Niacin, Sodium Selenite, Copper Gluconate, Pantothenic Acid, Manganese Sulphate, Vitamin A, Vitamin B6, Beta Carotene, Thiamin, Vitamin D, Vitamin B12 ,Riboflavin, Folic Acid, Biotin, Potassium Iodate*

In short, a sugared, artificially sweetened milk shake with the addition of chemically grown vitamins and minerals with added thickening agents to make you feel full – that's all it is.

Here is the list of ingredients for an ordinary chocolate milk shake:

Semi-skimmed Milk, Glucose Fructose Syrup, Sugar (3%), Fat Reduced Cocoa Powder (1%), Stabilisers: Cellulose, Cellulose Gum and Carrageenan, Natural Flavouring

When you compare the two drinks it is plain to see that, aside the addition of artificial sweeteners, vitamins and minerals, they are more or less the same. In fact, to be perfectly honest, the ordinary milk shake drink is probably better and has no artificial sweetener.

If I had to choose between the two, then I would choose the ordinary milk shake drink. Moreover, the human body does not assimilate well the artificial, chemically produced vitamins and minerals in this kind of pharmaceutical preparation.

But let's go ask your Granny! What would your Granny advise you to do here? Given the choice between an ordinary sensible meal and a sugared, artificially sweetened, artificially vitaminized and mineralized chocolate substitute drink, what would she advise?... Would she think that's healthy?... Do you think that's healthy?

The main question to ask yourself is what would you prefer? Do you really prefer to drink a bland concoction worthy of the best Shakespearean apothecary? When making your choice please bear in mind what happened to Romeo and Juliette! Or would you prefer to sit down to a nice, tasty meal where the heady aromas of cooking fill your home and your appetite?

Your wisdom already knows the answer to that. We are so brainwashed with dieting marketing images, combined with the simple desperation for a solution. A little bit of wisdom goes far in preventing us making, what ultimately could be, a terrible mistake.

Another point to bear in mind is that these substitute

drinks are nearly always based on sweet tasting milk shakes – chocolate, vanilla, strawberry, etc and yet, we are constantly told that we need to avoid those kinds of sweet beverages; for a company to be supposedly promoting weight loss and health through these products, it doesn't make much sense. There is a massive contradiction in the message, which is basically saying, "lose weight by eating the foods that are normally 'taboo' when we're dieting."

I followed one of these substitute meal plans myself in 1991, accompanying by a diet grape juice drink – I didn't lose any weight. However, in 1992 I ballooned up; my inner knowing is telling me that there is a correlation: that this product affected my metabolism, so that when I changed my diet the next year, through a change in circumstances, I didn't stand a chance!

Low-Fat Diets – Adipose Wrecks!

For several decades now, we have been told that for health reasons we must cut down our fat intake. After all, fat is responsible for heart disease, gallstones, hypertension, cholesterol. This is true, so it's a shame that fat tastes so good!

However, what we are not being told is how the fat is getting to the heart, the arteries, the kidneys... our hips! Yet, this is probably the most important piece of information that we need to know about how our bodies physically work so that we can lose weight and live healthily.

Here's your first clue Sherlock!
One of my relatives was recently diagnosed with gallstones and was immediately prescribed a low-fat diet. He's not allowed eggs, red meat, any fried food, any oils or anything containing cholesterol. However, he never was a big eater of fatty foods and actually has a fairly healthy diet; he has never had a problem with

weight gain, he is somebody that actually could be classed as underweight for his height, yet when he was just in his fifties he suffered a heart attack and has since been under medication – the famous cholesterol-reducing statins. Gallstones are directly related to high levels of cholesterol in the blood but my relative has been on statins for around seven years. So how is it that someone who has never eaten a high fat diet, who has never had a weight problem, and who has been on cholesterol-reducing statins for nearly a decade ends up with a heart attack and gallstones that are directly related to high levels of low-density cholesterol?

There is one thing that he is a big eater of and that is sugar. He's a "three-sugars-in-a-cup-of-tea" man, always has been and, most likely despite my nagging, always will be. He has a very "sweet tooth".

So what has sugar got to do with weight-gain, heart attacks and gallstones?

Elementary my dear Watson!

When we eat, different hormones and enzymes in our bodies jump into action to deal with the digestion and assimilation processes. One of those hormones is insulin, and one of the roles of insulin is to deal specifically with the levels of glucose in the blood. Easy to understand: when you eat a food that has a high sugar/starch content your body will produce more insulin than if you eat a food that contains a very low sugar/starch content in order to transform the sugar/starch into glucose.

However, along with the insulin production comes another process – lipogenesis. No need to be a Greek scholar to know that "genesis" is to do with the creation and "lipo" is to do with fat. So we are talking about the creation of fat cells - but here's the rub! Not only does this process of lipogenesis entail the storing of any fat content that you may have eaten, it also transforms the glucose into fat cells to be nicely stocked on all those parts of your body that inhibit your movements. And not only that! Through these processes the levels of LDL cholesterol and triglycerides increase – the higher the glucose content the higher the LDL and triglycerides will ultimately be. The sneaky part is that it's not immediately visible. Over time, you're heading for some serious fat-related problems but fat-related problems that are initially caused by sugar/starch.

There is a more in-depth explanation on the metabolic function of insulin that you will find in Part 3 of this book – *"The Practicalities of the Mind-Body Connection,"* under the section titled *"The Truth About the Glycemic Index."* And for specific scientific information there is an excellent one-hour documentary by the Dr. Robert Lustig - "Sugar, the Bitter Truth" - that you can easily find on YouTube and that I would highly recommend.

You may say, "Well, hold on a minute! Our bodies need glucose to run on!" Yes, that's true but it's only in the last hundred years or so that human beings have begun eating such large amounts of sugar and starch. Prehistoric man didn't need to quickly swallow a high glucose energy bar to give him that extra boost to help him run away from rampaging mammoths! The vast majority of us lead fairly sedentary lives and, through our technological and societal advances, we are perhaps even less active now than we have ever been in the history of man.

So what has this got to do with low-fat diets? At a first glance, given that insulin is responsible for stocking fat, you could say that it *would* be sufficient to cut down on the fat intake, but that alone will not hinder the lipogenesis process, nor be of any use in lowering the LDL cholesterol and triglycerides. As long as you continue to charge your body in glucose, an amount of glucose that the human organism is not designed to handle, those insulin-related processes will pursue unhinged.

Eating low fat serves absolutely no purpose whatsoever.

Now, of course I'm not saying to go out and have a fat food fest. I'm not saying don't cut off the fatty parts of meats or to not pay attention to our fat intake. What I am saying is that taking your diet to an excessively low fat regimen will neither solve the weight problems you may have, nor sort out any fat-related illnesses that you may be suffering from, it may in fact exacerbate them and even create other unpleasant metabolic problems. The main question to ask ourselves is, *"Is this what Nature intended for us?"*

In part two of this book we will deal with the reverse mechanism of how to lose weight and resolve the fat related health issues. And once more, I stress upon you that if you are under any kind of medicine related to diet/cholesterol/hypertension etc – you must continue to take that medicine until such times as your doctor and/or specialist advises you otherwise.

Designer Dieting

The latest diet in fashion! These are diets that are popular for a season or maybe even more. There's a whole lot of hype and marketing campaigns around them and then they quieten down and return into oblivion. These diets, like the latest Dior sunglasses, are designed to fit you for a moment in time. The authors of these diets are aware of that.
On the forums you will read enthusiastic reports from some and other reports from people who criticize them heavily after having tried and failed.
You also know that they are Designer diets because the content is not natural, they are diets that so obviously cannot be carried out over any length of time; many of

them are honestly presented as short-term quick-fix solutions.

Now, outside of any kind of efficiency brought by these diets, they are often restrictive and make socializing difficult, some can be extremely expensive and some can be excessive in their approach, rendering them dangerous. We must never forget that a thin waistline can be a gauge of health but is not a guarantee that what is going on inside our bodies is aligned with what would be an apparently healthy exterior.

These diets promise rapid results with little or no effort and while little or no effort is nice, when, for example, you're only allowed to eat one food group a day as some of these diets advise, after three days that can become quite an effort. Most of the time these diets are lacking in variety; variety of colour, variety of taste, not forgetting a variety of vitamins, minerals, oligo-elements - nutrients necessary for healthy body function. Often these diets will advise supplements in vitamins or other nutritive elements, which is clearly a sign that the diet is lacking in those elements. Others state that they will not take you on for "coaching" if you present certain medical conditions!

We need to wonder about these doctors and scientists who, despite their medical knowledge, promote diets that can in fact be dangerous for our health; though I do believe that in certain cases, even some of the extreme diets are created from a sincere place of caring for people and wanting to help them find a solution. But if you really want to help people, isn't it better to advise people on the natural way of eating that is not only good for them but will also help them lose weight – that is the goal of this book that you are reading.
Again, I am saying to you to be very careful with your choices – if it doesn't feel right, don't do it. If it sounds difficult to maintain, don't do it. If the diet carries

warnings, definitely don't do it. After years of trying out all of these different diets I came to the following conclusion, *"when in doubt, don't!"* And believe me, when you make your own decisions about what you want to put in your mouth and stomach, it's far easier to put a personal plan in place than following a set of guidelines that you don't, perhaps, quite understand the reason for.

As Supercoach Michael Neill says: *"You are the expert on you!"*

Hyper Protein Diets

These diets often fall into the category of "dissociated" dieting as they generally recommend eating only one food group per day, often animal protein, and cutting out any other kind of food substances. But, as Dr. Joe Leonardi author of "Obesity Undone" points out, if you only eat one food group cutting out all the rest then there's a good chance you will lose weight - but to what cost? These diets are efficient but they can also be highly dangerous and it's worth being vigilant.

The apparent efficiency of these diets is demonstrated through rapid weight loss with no sensation of hunger – you lose weight and you're not hungry! How fabulous is that? The metabolic mechanism of these diets is very simple; by only eating protein, be it animal protein or protein drinks, the pancreas is not solicited and therefore produces either very insignificant amounts of insulin or even none at all. I explained briefly weight gain with regards to insulin production. Here, very simply, the process is reversed and the body is obliged, as glucose is the "fuel" that our bodies run on, to draw from the reserves stocked in the fat cells. Basically, the fat cells are transformed into glucose to fuel the body, hence the weight loss. However, after a short period on this kind of diet, certain negative symptoms begin to appear. They may seem harmless, but have no doubt... they are not!

The lack of fibre in the diet induces constipation and, in some cases, severe constipation that can result in the intestine folding in on itself. The symptoms are abdominal pain, nausea, vomiting and rectal bleeding. In the most severe cases there can be serious complications such as intestinal necrosis and septicaemia.

Often these diets will recommend a large consumption of water and your body will most likely be screaming for water in order to aid the digestion of the protein and eliminate the constipation. The over-consumption of water, particularly when it is accompanied by a lack of essential nutrients, can lead to cerebral oedema, a condition similar to water on the brain, which in turn can lead to, after other unpleasant complications, central nervous system dysfunction resulting in seizures, brain damage, etc.

The imbalance of nutrients, due to the lack of variety in the diet, can lead to severe vitamin deficiency resulting in fatigue, lethargy, headaches, nausea, vomiting, blindness, scurvy, rickets, impaired blood coagulation, anaemia and a whole host of other vitamin deficiency related illnesses. Though you may not feel at all hungry, you are nevertheless suffering from malnutrition.

Another unpleasant and very common complaint linked to these diets is a bad case of halitosis. Now, halitosis is unfortunate in itself but, above all, it is a sign that something is wrong and here's why. Our bodies are programmed to produce insulin very naturally; it is a process that is supposed to happen when we eat. Now, these diets, as mentioned above, reverse the process entailing a very minimal or even non-existent insulin production. The body, being obliged to draw from the stored glucose in the fat cells, will break down the fatty acids resulting in a high concentration of ketones that in turn, lead to the production of acetone due to the decarboxylation of the ketone bodies. Prolonged use of these high-protein ultra low-carbohydrate diets, can produce ketosis, in which acetone is formed in body tissue. Ketosis, which is the prolonged excess of ketone bodies in the tissue and the blood leads in its turn to ketoacidosis.

Ketoacidosis is a pathological metabolic state where the pH of the blood undergoes a substantial decrease. In layman's terms, your blood turns acid, known in more simple terms as blood poisoning. Oddly enough, ketoacidosis is one of the main markers of type 1 Diabetes and oddly enough entails bad breath – the breath smells of nail varnish or paint thinner. Interestingly, acetone is an organic compound used in nail varnish and paint thinner. Before we go any further, ask yourself: would you deliberately ingest nail varnish or paint thinner?

On this kind of diet you are, in reality, forcing your body into a diabetic state. Diabetes is a debilitating illness that can result in blindness, stroke, gangrene and amputation, just to mention a few of the accompanying dangers. Untreated, diabetes results in ketoacidosis, due to the increased fat metabolism following the shortage of insulin. Do you want to put your body into a diabetic state?

This acidosis, blood poisoning, attacks all of the major organs in the body resulting in kidney and liver failure, brain damage, pulmonary arrest and heart failure – coma and death are the usual outcomes.

Obviously, these extreme health situations are due to unusually prolonged use of these diets with absolutely no medical support. Thankfully, most people stop these diets fairly rapidly; firstly due to the lack of variety, secondly due to the cost and, I believe, thirdly because somewhere deep down your Wisdom tells you, and your body tells you too, that it's not natural to eat in that manner.

You can never go far wrong when you use your own Wisdom.

Detox – Deceitful and Dangerous!

In recent years this kind of diet has seen a great expanse in its growth, whether it be through the beliefs people have around these diets or around the detox products that are more and more available. I think it is through our over sanitized society that these diets have seen such a great increase in their popularity; perhaps, also, through "over-abundance" and possible "over-indulgence" we believe that our bodies need to be purged and cleansed.

The very simple fact is that detox diets, in the manner that they are the most often carried out, are nothing more than starvation diets.

People will consume large quantities of water, herbal teas, thin soup or perhaps even a solitary diet of fruit, over a period ranging from a few days to several weeks, in the belief that they are doing something wonderful for their bodies when, in fact, they are depriving themselves of an array of vital nutrients. These diets now include different types of "treatment" gadgets: detox pills, pads, patches and various appliances – all guaranteed to rid us of those nasty toxins and poisons that roam around our bodies and blood stream!

These diets are based on the assumption that we have toxins or poisons in our bodies that we need to purge ourselves of, and that by doing so, we are going to feel more healthy and alive. These diets suggest that we will be doing our bodies a great favour by giving them a nice rest from all the rubbish we eat, our sedentary lives and our lack of exercise. The results will be apparent in our complexion and on our waistline. Our brains are going to think more clearly and we are going to feel energized. The simple fact is our bodies already, very naturally, eliminate any "toxins" through the liver and the kidneys. It's a wonderful, miraculous machine to be able to do that all on its own!

Just think about it: we can consume even to a dangerously huge quantity of alcohol (although definitely not recommended!) that is genuinely toxic, yet the body *can* eliminate it – though I daren't imagine the hangover! Even a person who has heavily overdosed *can* eliminate what are true toxins and survive; obviously in any severe life-threatening situation such as these, proper medical attention is obligatory and absolutely essential. The point is; if, as is claimed, our bodies were really full of harmful toxins, we would be ill.

Here are some of the problems related to this type of diet: The large consumption of liquids, going up to 3 or more litres of liquid a day, actually forces the kidneys and the liver into overtime. Your body, through the lack of food, finds itself in a state of hypoglycaemia, causing dizziness, headaches, nausea... Of course, the longer these detox diets are continued, the more you are exposing yourself to real health risks.

The question is: where, in all that, are we giving our bodies a rest?

A lot of the accompanying products for these detox diets come across as really quite gimmicky. They're often excessively expensive and often claim results that they don't actually produce. One example is the famous detox footbath. These footbaths claim to eliminate toxins through the soles of your feet, turning the water brown; a recent France 5 documentary showed that, once switched on, whether feet were present in the water or not, the water still turned brown through a simple process of oxidation. I'm not against footbaths; I think they can be very pleasant and relaxing. Again, a little Wisdom goes a long way to knowing whether a claim that is being made is honest or not.

The pills are just generally supplements in vitamins and minerals, which are not particularly well assimilated by the human body. Though there are no apparent health risk factors linked to these kinds of supplements, the long-term effects have still to be shown. Generally speaking, we can consider them to be harmless, though expensive.

The "detox holiday" now also exists. One such holiday beside the seaside, for a price ranging from 500€ to 2000€ per person, proposes the following two formulae:

Formula A	*Formula B*
Morning meditation	*Morning meditation*
Muscular exercises	*Muscular exercises*
Reflexology session	*Reflexology session*
(supplement)	*(supplement)*
Breakfast	*Breakfast*
– herbal teas/fruit juice	*– herbal teas/fruit juice*
A three-hour hike	*A three-hour hike*
Lunch -	*Lunch -*
more fruit juice and herbal tea	*a small bowl of wholemeal rice or vegetable juice or a small amount of raw food*

For both formulae the afternoon activities consist of either aesthetic care, including bowel irrigation or exercise including aerobics and spinning - on an empty stomach... Dinner for both formulae consists of a thin soup: for the formula B, there are mixed vegetables in the soup; for the formula A, it's just the stock.

I don't know about you but if I'm going to be spending money on a holiday beside the seaside, I'm going to expect fish and chips and ice cream after that three-hour hike! Those are foods that I don't eat on a very regular basis and, as one of my friend's father says, (who happens to be a top chef, Meilleur Ouvrier de France) "When you go somewhere special, eat the things that you wouldn't normally eat at home so as to make an occasion of it!" This gentleman has been known to serve up snake and lion in his restaurant; he definitely knows what out of the ordinary means!

The question to ask is: would you really enjoy a holiday like that? Practically no food, 3 hour hikes plus supplementary exercise, not forgetting the aforementioned optional bowel irrigation; given that most people only get between three to five weeks holiday a year – it sounds like quite an unpleasant waste of that valuable holiday time. Do you think your Granny would like a holiday like that?

My own Gran turned 90 a couple of years ago. Our family organized a holiday for her on the Orient Express – I think she thoroughly enjoyed it and as far as I know, the food, which consisted of three and four course meals, was delicious!

Diet Pills/Hunger Blockers

These pills come in various different forms, from concentrated vitamin supplements that promise the weight will magically fall away, to diet pills that carry strange, yet enticing names such as "carb blockers", "sugar blockers", "fat burners", "calorie burners", "insulin regulators", "muscle builders/body composition changers" and "appetite suppressants".

Some of these contain natural compounds. *All* of them promise results that you will *never* obtain. *All* of them are extremely expensive and *many of them* carry warnings that they should only be used on a short-term basis. One wonders what to do once you stop taking them?

The "natural" compound pills contain ingredients such as green tea, ginger, ginseng, ginko, different types of berries, citrus extracts, etc. Added to that, you will often find magnesium, manganese, chromium, folic acid, etc. plus additional vitamins, B group, vitamin C, etc.
But why take a pill with green tea extract when you can just drink green tea? – It actually tastes quite nice and if you add in a little lemon or mint, it can be a very refreshing drink. The point is, if you're eating cream cakes on a very regular basis, (and I'm not saying that you are, I'm just using this as an example) no amount of green tea extract is going to stop you putting on weight...

The only thing that a pill or tea can do is relieve your conscience, not much else. Somehow we're misled into believing that it's okay to eat "whatever" as long as we are taking the miracle pill. Often the publicity will claim just that: "Control your appetite, eat less calories and lose up to 5 pounds per week." Some carry false information on how the body works, stating that the factor in weight gain is a lack of energy and that our bodies oblige us to eat unhealthy foods that are high in energy – chocolate bars, sweets and high-calorie snacks; the publicity then goes on to claim that the magic remedy will boost the body's energy so that your body doesn't have the impression of a need for sweet foods. Allow me to take that apart: the feeling of lack of energy is coming from a state of hypoglycaemia, thus the desire for sweet foods. All of the foods mentioned contain high amounts of sugar.

A magic pill cannot boost the body's energy if, as the publicity claims, there is a lack of energy already present; the energy has to come from somewhere – that would be a little bit like expecting a lamp to work without plugging it into the electric current.

Unfortunately, if you don't know how your body works, it's very easy to be duped by this kind of publicity, and I'm speaking from experience.

A disclaimer that I found on the company website of one of these diet pills read as the following:

> "A diet pill that can in no way substitute any medication. The testimonials on this site are in no way representative of the recorded average weight loss. Each case is different and the weight loss for each person will vary depending on eating habits and exercise habits during the "cure" *Company Name* is not recommended for women who are pregnant and people suffering from any illnesses. For those suffering from an extreme weight problem, it is advised to consult your doctor. The testimonials presented here are sent in by consumers via e-mail or letter. While a minor percentage of consumers may perhaps lose a significant amount of weight in a short amount of time, this weight loss is not guaranteed for 100% of consumers."

The company's own disclaimer doesn't make the product sound particularly efficient.

The most disturbing, though, is that we are still maintaining the idea that we need to restrict ourselves, that we need to control ourselves and, in many cases, the publicity is designed to make us believe that without their magic solution, we will never attain the physical body that we dream of having... Ultimately, it just adds to the pressure that we already put upon ourselves.

Also, it's often difficult to find information on the full ingredients of these products. There are many controversial studies as to the benefits and adverse effects of these pills and I think it's really important to carefully consider before filling that glass of water; the pill may just be harder to swallow than imagined!

How much easier would it be to lose weight without all the extraneous thinking that we have about it? When we know that our weight, our physical appearance is not what our core being is really about, we can lose that sense of pressure, we can lose those thoughts and suddenly, what has been a weight problem becomes a weight solution. All it requires is a change in perspective, which is what we'll be discussing in Part 2 of this book.

Incidentally, I discovered that the best appetite suppressant that exists, the one that has existed since our planet formed, is food, the food provided by Mother Nature neither in pill nor potion form but real, natural food.

When Food Giants Become Food Ogres

In our society of abundance there have come to grow large food conglomerates that basically are in charge of the market.
Now, where that might not be such a bad thing as they give out employment and, for many of them, have found ways of making food "safer" and more available, there is, however, a big problem...

In the beginning, one person has the idea of making food available to as many people as possible – the idea in itself deserves much praise.

However, the more the company grows, the less human it becomes, the more it becomes greedy and the less it is concerned with the well being and health of the people it is supposed to be serving.

These are the people who can afford the big marketing

campaigns that play on our basic needs and instincts. I was listening to a conference recently where Michael Neill was speaking and he described the marketing model that is generally used in our society in the following manner. He puts it very nicely and with great humour:

> "Marketing at its worst! Tweak the insecure thinking of your reader or listener, which is not hard as we all have insecure thoughts, and then offer them relief in the form of your product or service. Satan's handbook for effective marketing!"

From a sales perspective that is "good" marketing, from a humane perspective, as Michael Neill points out, it's lacking in genuine love and we can sense that.

And it's true. That is what a lot of these big companies are doing. They look to where we feel weak and they attempt, through wonderful marketing images, to fill the gaps that we believe exist in our lives. And because we believe that, we blindly buy their products and then we are left with a bitter sensation wondering why George Clooney/Julia Roberts hasn't called yet begging for us to go out with them.

Now the marketing manipulation towards the public is one problem, the other problem is the utter control that these people have over the agro-business. These people, in order to make sure of huge profits, keep their thumb on the button whether it be at the governmental level, the scientific level or within the agro-business market itself.

Take some of the biggest companies who, in addition, have the monopoly on the market. They are willing to put our health on the line with modified, transformed, chemically produced products in order to protect their profit margin.

Many of the studies that come out claiming the health properties of certain foods – milk, sugar, wheat are a few examples – are financed by the Ogres themselves and the results are always in their favour. These biased studies are followed by huge marketing campaigns, leaning on the results of these self-financed studies, thus protecting their own sales and business. A lot of these companies have people within the government, passing bills, stating that foods are safe. When you look at the situation as a whole it can be really quite scary when you understand the level of manipulation – and all for financial profit.

For the most part of the population, we believe only what we are being told and therefore we carry on a lifestyle that can ultimately be harmful to our health. The risk for the companies is minimal. By the time the problems come to light, they will have changed strategies – the tobacco industry is perhaps one of the most flagrant examples of this. And so we shall have, bottles of milk carrying health warnings, sugary products similarly. Vegetables will carry labels stating that they were "grown with the use of pesticides" – and those will be the products that will be the most attractive pricewise and the people who will suffer the most from that will be those who are in the more unfortunate financial circumstances.

The companies, themselves, will be well protected, their argument will be that we were informed and forewarned.

But here's the thing. Their marketing campaigns play on our insecurities, but what if those gaps that you believe exist in your life, didn't exist – what if it was all just thought? If you think that something is missing, then you feel that something is missing. What if you didn't think and thus feel that? What would you do differently? Would you still buy their products?

I would like to treat just one last subject in this part of the book but that is not concerned so much by the restrictive element that can be found in other diet solutions – the organic market.

Organic Food – the Good, the Bad and the Swindle

The Good

I think we all agree that organic food is better for our health. The organic market is highly regulated as far as GMOs, pesticides, herbicides, antibiotics and pesticides are concerned and, while there is much controversy over the long-term effects of these substances, that are designed to increase production and ensure sales, again I always say *"when in doubt, don't!"*

Organic food tastes better and often has a more natural aspect. In my local organic shop, the ham they sell is not lush pink, it is grey, because there is no colouring – that says a lot about the amount of colouring that must be in the general products that are on sale in the super- and hypermarkets. It makes you wonder about the long-term impact on health.

From a practical point of view, the shops are smaller and, once you are used to going there and know which products you are going to buy, your shopping is done more rapidly and, in general, these places tend to smell nice when you go in – you can smell the wholeness.
A lot of the time the produce is local, which is a better guarantee of preserved vitamins, minerals, etc and also guarantees less manipulation of the product, cooling, freezing, forced maturation...

Organic produce is generally grown with respect to the Earth and Nature: crop rotation, allowing the soil to rest and regenerate between harvesting and re-seeding, and planting seasonal produce, thus avoiding exhausting the goodness in the land.

The local produce will have been picked when ripe, which is interesting not only from an environmental point of view but also because they are complete from a nutritional point of view.

The Bad

I think the biggest problem people have when it comes to organic produce and organic food is the pricing. Some of the products are exceedingly expensive and, if you're on a smaller budget and/or have a family to feed, eating organic does not always seem like a good solution financially speaking. Many of us would like to buy these products because we know that they are more natural but the price puts us off.

I have actually been doing a few experiments with regards to this. Now, I myself eat a fairly basic diet, and thus so does my family as I'm the head chef in the kitchen! I have done a few comparisons as far as pricing is concerned, that can be quite surprising.

I found that by buying just the basics that my weekly shopping doesn't actually come to very much more than what I would have normally paid in the supermarket. There is at the most a 10€ difference in price which is not huge when you think about the nutritional and environmental advantages.

I think that as organic shops are smaller, there is less choice and this "lack" of choice means that I'm only buying the items that we actually need, there is less to tempt us. I go with my shopping list and replace the missing items in my fridge and cupboards.

The "downside" to buying just the basics, is that you have to make food from scratch and in our busy society of today that can feel like a rather arduous task. After a long day at work, when you're getting home and you're tired, it's not always easy to start getting the chopping board out and to start preparing food for a meal.

The other disadvantage is that, in the organic food stores, we may not find all of the products that we need. For example, my local organic shop doesn't sell bin bags or washing powder. That means that I have to do my shopping in several different places, which can be time consuming. That being said, when I have to go to the supermarket or another type of shop for the items that I can't find, I usually will buy them in bulk, to avoid returning too often.

The Swindle

A lot of people believe, and I believed this myself at one point, that by simply eating organic it is possible to lose weight and be 100% healthy. I have to admit, that is the marketing image that is sold to us, though perhaps not explicitly.

Now, eating basic foods will be a help but take a visit round your local organic shop and you will find similar kinds of transformed products on the shelves – yes, the ingredients will be mostly organic but if the first ingredient on the label is sugar, it doesn't make much difference to your waistline and your health whether it's organic or not. So, if you go to your organic shop and you carry on buying the same transformed type foods that you would normally have bought in the supermarket, you are not going to lose weight.

You will also find in these shops the usual array of vitamin supplements, substitute meals along with a panoply of diet pills, designed, as the images and information on the packaging tell us, to make or help us lose weight. Yes, a lot of these are based on organic compounds but my point is, there is no magic pill. The real solution is to change your eating habits. By all means, if you wish to take supplements in vitamins that are organically based, then do so – again, I'm not here to tell you what to do or what not to do. But it seems to me a very expensive solution to a need that can be easily covered in your daily diet just by eating normally, particularly if your buying local organically and seasonal produced goods.

The other inaccuracy concerning organic food that many of us are not aware of, is organically labelled food doesn't have to be 100% organic. Some is, but some contain substances that are not found in the organic production chain.

The other worry, though far less apparent, is that Genetically Modified Foods (GMOs) are beginning to infiltrate even the organic industry, chiefly in the form of corn and soya. In the States, it's not always obligatory to label if a food is GMO, or if meat comes from an animal that received GMO feed. It's important to know that if you want to be 100% sure, you have to buy 100% organic. Only a **100% organic label** guarantees that the final product does not contain genetically modified ingredients in some form or another.

Also important to bear in mind is that an organic farmer, who has a non-organic farmer neighbour, will experience the pesticides and chemicals from the non-organic farmer being carried into his organic fields via the wind, insects, pollination and soil infiltration.

Another important point; some organic farmers, though using sustainable methods of farming and producing organic food, can find themselves exempt from the organic labelling if they are unable to attain a certain annual income from the sales of their produce – that does seem a little unfair for those who are making an effort to take care of the planet and its inhabitants.

Lastly, I would just like to give my own personal opinion on this. Now, I realize that there has been an enormous amount of change in agricultural production but my Granny had never heard of organic. Previously, we didn't need labelling to know what was right or not to eat.

There is, in all honesty, quite a lot of controversy around whether organic food is healthier and whether it really contains more vitamins than the more general produce that we can find in the supermarket. From my own personal point of view, I don't much like man-made chemicals. My choice in eating organic, when I do so, is based on the fact that I wish to be exposed, and expose my family, as little as possible to artificial chemical compounds.

As I say, we eat a very basic diet: one my Granny would have been happy to eat!

The Truths Behind Food – What We Don't See

In this first section of the book we have discussed the problematic of the diet market and some of its implications, many of which are unhealthy and some of which can even be dangerous.
In this section, I would like to discuss with you the true value of food and why some of the foods that we buy, that appear healthy, are perhaps not as good for us as we are led to believe. In a sense it's a continuation of what we have already discussed, with more detail on specific food groups.

However, there are a certain number of physiological mechanisms going on in your body that, if you are not aware of the true value of food and what is really in it and how that affects our metabolism, then you may be making, as I did, superhuman efforts and not getting anywhere without really knowing why.
Once more the idea is to become aware of what we are doing; what we are putting into our systems so that we can make the right choices for ourselves and not just blindly follow this or that recommendation.

What the Word "Diet" Really Means

The word diet has its origins in Latin and Greek. The ancient meaning of the word was "an assembly/a council" that would meet on a daily basis. It also meant "a way of living." The Greek word meant, "to lead one's life." It also meant "a day's work" or "a day's salary/allowance" In the early 13th century the word was used to indicate "regular food."

It is only from the 14th Century onwards that the word took on a restrictive connotation and has only been used with the meaning that we imply today since the mid 1600s, which you will agree is fairly recent.

When we take the word "diet" back to its original meaning, then it simply means your daily dose of food. It's interesting to note that, before the invention of money, people would be paid with food for their families – you could call it the original gold (chicken) nugget!

It's ironic to note that previously, in times when food could be scarce and even non-existent, that the term meant "regular food." In contradiction, we have now what can only be described as an over-abundance of food and the word has become symbolic of "restriction" – how times can change!

If you were to consider a diet as simply something you do on a daily basis without the involvement of restriction in any manner – what would you do? How would you eat? What would you change, if anything?

Many people are afraid that if they didn't make up the rules around what they are supposed to eat or not eat, they would just eat "junk" the whole time. This simply is not true. Sure, you might do that for a few days, maybe even a few weeks, but your body would very quickly start giving you signs that this is not what it wants or requires.

Of course, the problems arise when we don't listen to our bodies and don't pay attention to our food requirements as a "way of living." Unfortunately for some, the available information is so confusing that we continue to eat badly and end up suffering the physiological and the psychological consequences of those unhealthier eating habits but even then, if we can tune into our bodies, we will quickly become aware of what we really require food wise.

In 2004, the American actor and documentary filmmaker, Morgan Spurlock, took on the challenge to eat food at a famous fast food chain and only food from that famous fast food chain. For a whole month, breakfast, lunch and dinner was eaten at this chain and the experiment was documented in the film Supersize Me! The film is well worth the watch if you haven't seen it. It is as entertaining as it is informative.

On the second day of the experiment, Mr. Spurlock, who leads normally a fairly healthy lifestyle, has been "supersized" in the restaurant chain. The result is simple to understand – he vomits the lot, everything that he's eaten. The body, not being made to cope with such huge doses of junk, rejects it.

However, as the month goes on, his body not only "adapts" to this "diet" but begins craving it. Outside of the physical consequences, and we're talking liver damage, kidney problems, hypercholesterolemia, heart problems; there are also psychological effects. He starts to feel irritable and jumpy. He finds himself in a low state of mind that can only be "fixed" by the fast food.

Interestingly, these are some of the signs that your body gives out when it's trying to tell you that it doesn't want to comply with what you're eating; that's it's not able to assimilate what you are putting in and that it needs something different, dare I say, something better.

Of course, this is an extreme example – very rare are the

people who actually force themselves to have such a bad diet over such long periods of time, but even in small doses, your body will react and let you know. If you listen to your body you will be able to put into place what it really needs, what YOU really need, without any effort, without actually having to think about it.

Now if you're unsure of what your body needs and it's true, after many years of unintuitive eating habits we don't always know instinctively what we need, we have forgotten somewhat how to listen to our bodies, there is a simple experiment that you can do, one that I teach my clients.

Focus on one food group or one food, for example an avocado.
Don't eat that food for a certain amount of time. That can be going from several days to even several weeks. Do eat it if you start to crave it within the time period, if you're craving it that means your body needs it. More precisely that means that your body requires something that is in the avocado. After your decided time period, even if you don't have a craving for it, eat one and record the effect that it has on your body, how you feel physically and emotionally. If anything is amiss then, very simply that food is not right for you.

A female client used this experiment to monitor the effects of a certain food on her body. She chose to start with milk. For two weeks she abstained from drinking milk, then for two days in a row she drank a bowl of milk in the morning. She reported back that she felt bloated and quite nauseated. She decided not to drink milk again as she wanted to listen to, and do what she felt was intuitively right for her body.

A personal example of the same thing, which provoked quite a lot of hilarity amongst my friends, was a sudden craving that I got for Brussels sprouts – the hilarity was mostly provoked by the misplaced reputation carried by Brussels sprouts at the end of their digestive process! I ate around two pounds of Brussels sprouts that day, lightly steamed and salted out of a bowl in much the same way as I might have eaten a bowl of potato chips. Whatever is in the Brussels sprouts, that day I was in need of it and my body informed me of it via the craving. I also knew that it was right by the feeling of increased energy and vitality that I experienced in the following hours and days.

A more obvious example of this are the cravings women have during pregnancy. As this is a case of not only the survival of the woman but also of the tiny baby growing inside the womb, the cravings feel stronger and can be extremely impulsive, leading to some rather humorous mixings of food and also some rather repulsive mixings of food! No matter, the body is simply crying out for what it needs and all we have to do is simply listen and respond to that need. It's that simple!

So if we really do want to be on a diet, we can do so but in the manner that it was originally intended – i.e. "a way of living" "leading a life" "regular food" – giving our bodies on a daily basis what they really require to survive in the healthiest manner possible.

The Importance of Reading Food Labels

When I first started out doing this, some fifteen to twenty years ago, I used to drive anybody that dared come shopping with me completely up the wall. My shopping trips could last anything from one to up to four hours.

Like many people, I used to make a shopping list, dash round to the shops, grab what I "needed" from the shelves, throw it in the basket, run to the checkout, shove the goods in the carrier bags, get home as quickly as possible, pack away the goods (or the bads) into the cupboards and fridge, breathe a huge sigh of relief and finally sit down with a nice cup of tea and a chocolate biscuit.

I used to do that, not any more! (Okay, I admit I still sometimes do the cup of tea and chocolate biscuit at the end)

It started out as simple curiosity: I just wanted to know what was in the food that I was buying but I became more astonished and even shocked at what I saw. Here is one of my favourite examples:

Example 1
Chicken Breast (65%), Bread Crumb, Vegetable Oil, Wheat Flour, Water, Salt, Maltodextrin, Stabiliser (Trisodium Citrate), White Pepper, Potato Starch, Yeast Extract, Citrus Fibre, Acidity Regulator (Sodium Carbonate), Whey Powder, Garlic Extract, Bread Crumb contains: Wheat Flour, Yeast, Salt, Dextrose, Emulsifier (Mono- and Di-Acetyltartaric Esters of Mono- and Di-Glycerides of Fatty Acids), Vegetable Oil, Antioxidant (Ascorbic Acid)

Example 2
Cereals, Meat and Animal Derivatives (including 4% Chicken), Vegetable Protein Extracts, Oils and Fats (0.25% Fish Oil, 0.1% Sunflower Oil), Derivatives of Vegetable Origin, Minerals (including 0.2% Sodium Tripolyphosphate), Vegetables (4% Carrots, 4% Peas), Antioxidants, Colorants from Natural Origin

They look fairly similar, don't they?...

The first is **chicken nuggets** that we give liberally to our children and at times eat ourselves. The second... well the second is **cat food**!... Bon appétit!

Now you understand, with a rather extreme example, why I check the labelling on the packaging and why I nearly never buy chicken nuggets.

What shocked me most were the long lists of ingredients, largely unpronounceable and for the most part, unless you happen to have a scientific background in chemistry, incomprehensible. In time, however, they started to make sense. What I quickly realized was that these strange ingredients were added to the food for five main reasons: to thicken, to replace something else, to enhance the flavour, to render the aspect more appetizing and to preserve.

As it dawned on me that food didn't naturally contain all those mysterious added ingredients, I consciously made the decision to only buy foods that contained a maximum of three ingredients, apart from the odd exception and I have to admit that I very rapidly started to notice a difference health wise. Physically, I noticed that I was less agitated, sleeping better and feeling generally more energized. I was more awake during the day, certainly also because the sleeping had improved, and I was able to concentrate better on the tasks that I had to accomplish during the day. Psychologically, I had less mood swings.

With the improvement in my feeling of health, I took things to a further level and consciously made the decision to only buy foods with one ingredient. I'm exaggerating slightly but it was from then that my eating habits returned to basics and, oddly enough, my shopping bill was much less expensive. When I go to the supermarket now, I only visit three or four aisles and one of those is for the cleaning products. Of course living in France, I will occasionally make a detour to the wine department, it's mandatory here otherwise you lose your residence permit, at least that's my excuse!

I want to be clear. When I'm talking about reading the food labels I am not talking about the GDA (Guideline Daily Amount) or, as they have in some shops in Great Britain now, the traffic light system. Unfortunately these particular labels can lure us into a sense of false assurance. As long as what is on the label enters into the

GDA or the traffic light is mostly green, then we feel safe in buying those products. They are there, supposedly, to simplify the buying process, to make it easier for the consumer to understand what he or she is buying - I believe, and I'm not alone in this, that they are there for marketing purposes and so that we don't ask too many questions.

When I am talking about reading food labels, I'm talking about the fine print, the actual ingredients. You may have a green traffic light on the packaging but in the product have artificial sweeteners and chemical additives that you may not want to consume it.

Entire books have been written with the lists and explanations of all the chemical ingredients that go into our food nowadays – entire books! The list is long going from modified starch, thickening agents, added vitamins to the thousands of mysterious E numbers that may or may not have a natural origin and for many of them, the natural origin leaves a lot to be desired – bugs and beasties and stuff, oh my! We also should bear in mind that the producers are not obliged to notify us of everything that is present in the final product – many a time we are consuming ingredients without even knowing it.

The main question that I would suggest you ask yourself is, "Do you want what you eat to be controlled by another entity or do you want to make up your own mind?"

My solution of buying the basics, fruit and vegetables, grains and pulses, meat, fish and eggs means that I am sure, more or less, of what I'm actually buying and putting on my plate.

Again, I'm not telling you what to do but I'm asking you to think about it and decide what you believe to be best for you.

A recent Daily Mail article that I had the immense pleasure of reading and that was really very informative explained that some weird and wonderful ingredients found their way into our food products, here is a shortlist. Important to note that these are FDA approved:

Rat hair in chocolate, **crushed beetles** in drinks, the **anal secretion and urine** of beavers, **fish bladder**, **sheep's wool** (to be honest, sheep's wool seems a lesser evil than beaver butt!), **duck feathers**, **toilet bleach**, **sawdust**, **maggots**, **sand** and **pig skin**!

> *"I'll have the duck feathers with maggots and crushed beetles please, and a side order of sawdust. Just a little toilet bleach though, I don't want to overdo it on the sauce!"*

Sure makes finding a caterpillar on the salad seem less dramatic! This reminds me of a joke we told when I was a little girl:
"What's worse than finding a worm in an apple?"
"Finding half a worm!"
The difference of course is that in the apple you can see the worm, or the bit that's left, and decide whether to eat it or not. When it's crushed into our food and disguised as something else, you are eating it unknowingly.

Healthy Means More Expensive? – Not Necessarily!

It is noticeable that the "healthier" a food product, the more expensive it is. This poses an enormous problem when you are living on a small budget and have perhaps several mouths to feed.
The saddest story I ever read was about a family who were buying their food in a low cost supermarket. They had bought beef burgers that were contaminated (with e-coli I believe) and their baby died from food poisoning.

Is this the society that we really want to live in? Where the poorer amongst us are obliged to take risks with their health and even their lives in order to feed themselves? I would like to believe that our society would have evolved since the dark ages but certain aspects leave a lot to be desired.

We have industrial farming, battery hens, intensive fish farming, the mindless mass killing of animals for food; pesticides, herbicides, transformed foods, genetically modified foods, chemical additives. The technological advances in our Western civilization should allow us to produce safe food for everyone on the planet but, for profit, we are rendering our food unsafe and unhealthy. We consume and discard. We behave as if today is going to last forever, as if the planet's resources were going to last forever, and we do not respect them.

The extinction of animals has increased at an exponential rate in this last century; the bees that are necessary for our own survival are suffering and dying out, something that has never been seen on this earth before other than through extreme natural disasters, but this time we are the cause of that due to our mindless parasitic behaviour. I believe that we are the worst predator that the earth has ever seen for we use the resources and when there is a surplus, instead of dealing with it efficiently, we throw it away.

We are destroying the environment and the climate and for no good reason – we are neither taking care of the earth's survival, nor of our own.

But I do believe that each of us, individually, can take action. If we don't buy the products, or at least buy less of them, then the big companies that are controlling the industry will have no choice but to change their ways, but for the moment the score stands: Food Industry – 1 People Power – not much!

I remember being in Sunday school and playing a game with our teacher where we picked out flags representing different countries around the world. I got the United States; others got Britain, China, Africa, etc. Our teacher then proceeded to give us rolls of bread, the amount being based on the country that we had. As the United States, I got nearly all the bread rolls. At the time there was a famine in Africa, so Africa didn't get any. The teacher then asked us what we wanted to do, how we thought best to deal with the situation and so I shared out what I had, so that we all had an equal amount. I've done this same game with my own children, with the same results.

If a child can work that out, why is it that we as adults cannot?

To come back to food pricing, I have found that by buying basic food, by doing the cooking from scratch, just as my grandmother and even my mother did, that I am able to feed my family successfully with a very reasonable budget without having to resort to low cost supermarkets where the food, to be honest, is full of crap! I even manage fairly frequently to buy organic produce: the trick is to make sure that it is in season when it can be practically the same price as the non-organic produce and even, on the odd occasion, less expensive.

Yes, I daresay we eat a little differently than other families, I will make dishes that will last for several days, and I will make soups from the leftovers. We do occasionally buy foods that are processed and refined, but those are the exception to the rule. I alternate between meals that have a more expensive basis and meals that are super cheap. Yes, it requires a certain organization and certainly a bit of time but, in all honesty, when I have a stew in the oven that is going to cook for four hours, I don't have to do anything, it cooks all by itself. I then have four hours to do my work or anything else that I want or need to do.

The Light Food Lie

When I still consumed milk products I had got into the habit of buying a 0% fat yoghurt, produced by Danone called "Taillefine" – "thin waist". I had been happily eating my yoghurts for quite some time and really quite enjoyed them until one day I noticed something odd, something different. The yoghurt appeared to be creamier and thicker, the texture had changed and so had the taste, which was frankly a little bland. Intrigued by this new aspect, I was curious to know what they had changed in the product to make it like that. Unfortunately, I had thrown the cardboard packaging away so had to wait till the next visit to the shops.

Here's what I discovered: Danone, in order to make the yoghurt have this creamier aspect, had added modified starch and gelatine to thicken it up.

The advertising leads you to believe that these yoghurts are healthy and will help you lose weight but modified starch is a high GI carbohydrate that will provoke a high insulin release and the consequential lipogenesis that we already discussed.

One thing that is significant and really should be taken into account with regards to anything that is low fat, low-sugar, light, etc. is the amount of chemical additives that can be found in these products. There is much debate on the effects of chemical additives and the famous "e" numbers. Many believe that they are carcinogenic, that they can cause visual and auditive troubles, nervosity, brain cell damage and psychological problems such as depression and worse through the effect on the brain and body chemistry.

I'm not a scientist and there are many conflicting studies on the subject so I use my time-old adage, "if in doubt, don't!" Again, this is my own "rule of thumb", I'm not saying you have to make it yours...

The truth behind the low-fat produce is that in order for it to be appetizing from the viewpoint of texture, aspect and taste, the producers will add in whatever is necessary to do that. The worst for me in this is that, to come back to food labelling, if you only base your purchase on the GDA or traffic light system, then you are being horribly misled. The GDA on these products looks good, the traffic light is green across the board, yet you are buying and consuming a product that is NOT healthy.

So, again, I keep it very simple. If I buy cream, I buy full cream. Whatever I'm buying will be in its most natural form possible. If I buy a product that has sugar in it, or if I'm going to make something at home that requires sugar, then I use real sugar. I know what the consequences on my body will be and I know how to deal with that. For me the most important is to be aware of the effect, not so that we can make a ton of rules about it but so that we have more liberty in our choices. Personally, I am not willing to fool my body and mislead it into a state where, physically, it doesn't know what to do or how to react.

In the past, people ate sugar, people ate cakes, and people ate fat. At the same time they also ate a very basic daily diet and were, to all accounts and purposes, in better health than we are now.

Sugar Shame

We spoke previously about reading food labels and the long lists of ingredients that go into our food products. One important thing to know is that the ingredients are listed from the largest amount to the smallest amount on the packaging.
Now, if you're buying something very basic then that isn't really a problem, where the problems start is when

you are buying elaborate industrially manufactured products.

Here are a few examples of foods that we eat at breakfast and as snacks:

Wholegrain Cereals:
Wholegrain Wheat (93%), Sugar, Malt Extract (from Barley), Partially Inverted Sugar Syrup, Salt, Niacin, Iron, Pantothenic Acid, Vitamin B1 (Thiamin), Vitamin B2 (Riboflavin), Vitamin B6, Folic Acid, Vitamin B12.

When we read the titling "wholegrain wheat" we automatically assume that the product is healthy. On closer inspection we quickly discover that the second ingredient is sugar, the third ingredient 'malt' is also sugar, followed by a fourth ingredient, which is also sugar. To take away the overly sweet taste, salt is added and then we have a bunch of artificially fabricated added vitamins.

Crunchy Nut Cornflakes:
Maize, Brown Sugar (Sugar, Molasses), Peanuts (7%), Sugar, Honey (2%), Barley Malt Flavouring, Salt, Vitamins & Minerals: Niacin, Iron, Vitamin B6, Vitamin B2 (Riboflavin), Vitamin B1 (Thiamin), Folic Acid, Vitamin B12.

The first ingredient is corn, which has a very high GI, particularly through the processing that it goes through in order to make the cereal. Second ingredient sugar and don't be misled by the word brown – brown sugar does not have a lower GI than white sugar, third ingredient peanuts, but only 7%, fourth ingredient more sugar, fifth ingredient honey which is a sugar, fifth ingredient barley malt which is sugar, again the salt to remove the overly sweet taste and the added vitamins.

And a popular one for children, **Rice Krispies**:
Rice, Sugar, Salt, Barley Malt Flavouring, Niacin, Iron,

Vitamin B6, Riboflavin (B2), Thiamin (B1), Folic Acid, Vitamin B12.

It's nothing more than a big bowl of sugar! The rice is refined and "popped," giving it a very high GI. Sure, there are a few added, artificially manufactured vitamins but a healthy cereal that does not make. It's small wonder that our dear little cherubs are tired and irritable mid-morning, craving sweet foods and having trouble concentrating until lunchtime. They then will eat a lunch that is often comprised of foods containing sugar and/or a high starch content and exactly the same thing will happen mid-afternoon. If it happens that the teacher is also subjecting him/herself to a similar style of diet, this can explain a lot about the serious problems that can arise within the classroom.

And did you know that sugar is addictive? There are two main reasons for that. The first is precisely to do with the insulin production and the subsequent low blood sugar. As previously explained, the higher the GI, the higher the peak in the blood glucose levels and the lower the subsequent blood sugar will be. It seems fairly obvious that if you have a very low blood sugar, you're going to be craving something very sweet, something with a very high GI, to fill the gap. And so the process repeats itself ad infinitum. Just as a reminder, some of the signs of a low blood sugar are irritability, difficulty concentrating, tiredness, shakiness, blurred vision, tinnitus and dizziness.

The other reason sugar is so addictive is that it releases endorphins in the brain, in much the same way as cigarettes do. In a similar fashion to the insulin mechanism, following the initial endorphin release, there is a subsequent endorphin dip, which again provokes cravings for sweet/high GI items.

As our bodies become "accustomed" to the sugar or

glucose intake, we then find that the endorphin release is not as important as when we started out, which is to say that the glucose doesn't induce the endorphin release that our bodies have become used to. The endorphin release becomes resistant to the glucose intake and therefore we end up consuming more and more sugar/high GI foods in order to achieve those "happy" feelings that our bodies are awaiting through the endorphin release. That's what I call a sweet, vicious circle.

Looking at these examples of breakfast cereals, what is striking is the need for the added vitamins. The refining processes of the raw ingredients deplete them of all their natural goodness. Without the added vitamins you may as well just eat cardboard, in fact I think you may find more vitamins in the cardboard!

Is the amount of sugar that goes into these products really necessary, especially when followed by the addition of salt to remove the sickly sweet taste? The mixing of salt and sugar is a long-used technique to make the food we eat seem more appetizing. The mixture of the two opposing tastes makes us salivate more and the salivation, as everyone knows, is the first step in the process of digestion, that part of the digestive process that makes you actually want to put the food in your mouth.

The mixture of sugar and salt also makes the food tastier and make us more likely to want to eat more of it. How many of us have had a bowl of this type of cereal and gone back for a second one because it "just tastes so good?"

Strawberry Jam:
Glucose-Fructose Syrup, Strawberries, Sugar, Citric Acid, Gelling Agent: Pectin; Acidity Regulator: Sodium citrate; Strawberry Concentrate.

Sugar!... With a bit of fruit!

Some jams are made uniquely with the fruit and the sugar with roughly 50% of each ingredient going into the finished product. A famous French label of jam indicates 50g of fruit per 100g with 60g sugar per 100g – 50g plus 60g equals 110g!

I actually make my own jam in my bread machine. In fact all you need is the fruit and the pectin, which jellifies the fruit.

In the olden days making jam with the sugar was a way of preserving the fruit that would otherwise have gone bad. Many of the preserving techniques that we use today have their origins in the past when it was necessary to store food during the winter months. The problem is that today, the preservation techniques have gone off the scales and the scarcity of food, at least in Western society, is no longer a problem.

What's really scary is that the GDA looks good on the product and the traffic light system is 80% green! Why? Because it has fruit in it? Come on!

Ask yourself this. Would you take a strawberry, weigh it, weigh out the equivalent in sugar and a bit more and then eat the two together? How sick do you think that might make you feel? Would it feel natural to do that? After all, strawberries are sweet enough on their own.

For me the worst case is a famous chocolate-hazelnut spread that we give liberally to our children on bread or toast. Here are the ingredients:

> *Sugar, Vegetable Oil, Hazelnuts (13%), Fat-Reduced Cocoa (7.4%), Skimmed Milk Powder (6.6%), Whey Powder, Emulsifier (Soy Lecithin), Vanillin.*

The first ingredient is sugar; the second is oil with **only 13% of hazelnuts and 7.4% cocoa**. When you watch the publicity for this particular product, the images flow past of a fountain of "healthy" milk with a rainstorm of hazelnuts all mixed in with a tornado of yummy-healthy chocolate. The publicity presents it as a healthy food item, necessary for a child's growth and well being; you can see yourself from the list of ingredients that that could not be further from the truth.

And it's the same across the board. Take any industrially manufactured food product and you will find similar lists of ingredients. When we compare wholemeal bread to white bread, we quickly see that there is very little difference in the quality of the ingredients but we are continuously misled, by clever marketing campaigns, into believing that what we are consuming is healthy.

I remember once my mother seeing the diabetic dietician at the hospital who basically said that there was no need for her to only ever eat wholegrain bread and that eating the white bread was just the same – the dietician knew that and that's going back nearly twenty years! What saddens me is that she didn't say to my mother that, given her condition, she would be best to avoid bread altogether, at least the industrially manufactured kind.

Some of the publicity is more honest and can even be very entertaining. Take for example the famous Twix bar, of which the ingredients are:

> *Sugar, Glucose Syrup, Wheat Flour, Vegetable Fat, Skimmed Milk Powder, Cocoa Butter, Cocoa Mass, Milk Fat, Whey Powder, Lactose, Fat Reduced Cocoa, Salt, Emulsifier (Soya Lecithin), Raising Agent (E500), Natural Vanilla Extracts, (Traces: Hazelnut, Almond).*

If you ever get a chance to check out the commercials on YouTube, you will have a lot of fun, they are quite hilarious. Here's one of my favourites:

> *"Don't ask what are you going to do today? But what aren't you going to do today?*

Don't ask what is in a Twix? But what isn't in a Twix? (Jings, they're afraid we might find out!!!)
There's chewy caramel – rich milk chocolate – and that great cookie crunch!
Life's too interesting for a snack that isn't!"

Well, even though we know that it's not healthy and they know that it's not healthy, you have to admit that the advertising is ingenious and not misleading. The ingenuity also comes from the fact that by making the ad entertaining we associate a certain feeling with regards to the product which, that in itself, makes us want to buy it.

A few years back a famous coffee producer ran a long-term commercial series. It was basically a romantic story between this very sophisticated and beautiful lady and her hunk of a neighbour. The basic storyline was the fact that they were always on the verge of getting it on but never quite crossing the threshold, and this ad went on for years with people actually tuning in and catching up on the story, waiting avidly for the next instalment – fabulous marketing, completely playing on our romantic ideals and emotions and completely capturing the audience and thus, the consumer.
Whether you agree with them or not, you have to admire the people that came up with that.

However, this next one is particularly deceptive, a product that we give our children believing, through the publicity, that we are giving them something that is not only tasty but full of goodness:

Kinder chocolate:
Fine Milk Chocolate 40% (Sugar, Whole Milk Powder, Cocoa Butter, Cocoa Mass, Emulsifier: Soy Lecithin; Vanillin), Sugar, Skimmed Milk Powder, Vegetable Fat, Concentrated Butter, Emulsifier (Soy Lecithin), Vanillin, Total Milk Solids: 33%, Total Cocoa Solids: 13%.

The spiel on the product is the following and I have bolded the most shocking parts – what do you think?

"Designed for kids (!!!)

Small child-sized portions (!!!)

High quality ingredients (sugar is not a high quality ingredient)

Full of milky goodness (33% does not fullness make)

Perfect as a little treat! (!!!)

Fine milk chocolate bar with a delicious milky filling, Kinder Chocolate is perfect as a little treat or snack! Great care is taken in making sure that only the highest quality ingredients make it into our products.

*Kinder is of course the German word for children. Kinder Chocolate was the first Kinder product to be launched in the world, introduced in Germany over 40 years ago. Literally **invented for kids**, Kinder set new standards for chocolate, developing little Mini Treats bars in a "kinder"-size portion.*
*The launch of the Snack Bar format followed 20 years later, to enjoy the distinctive Kinder Chocolate taste in a format **more suitable for older children**.*
*Both Kinder Chocolate Mini Treats and Snack Bars were fully introduced in the UK and Ireland in 2001. Each year they are going from strength to strength as **mums become increasingly familiar with the great taste of Kinder Chocolate**.*

*100g of Kinder Chocolate contains the most important nutritional elements (proteins, calcium and **some vitamins**) of 250ml of milk. Milk contributes towards children's growth and helps to maintain **healthy food habits**. Kinder Chocolate's milk is carefully selected following strict criteria with regard to origin, quality and processing."*

In short, a bar of sugar and fat specially designed for children that is being passed off as **necessary** for creating "healthy food habits" among our youngsters with the publicity directly targeting mothers who are desperate to ensure that their child or children get the best out of life. I don't swear very often but that one, in particular, makes me want to swear or at least vociferate vehemently.

However, what shocked me the most was discovering that in the French "Plan National Nutrition Santé" (PNNS) – National Plan for Nutrition and Health, which was put in place by the French government as a means of containing and fighting against the growing obesity problem in this country, it is written that for a snack it is recommended to give a child "a chocolate bar such as a Kinder." This national plan is the one that is widely used among the medical profession and nutritionists in France and in which the everyday man and woman places their faith and their nutritional choices for their children and themselves.

The truth of the matter is that this plan, although requested by the government, was largely financed by the food conglomerates, and the majority of the scientists and nutritionists involved in the study happen to be on those food conglomerates' payrolls!

The twists in this system are fully documented in Thierry Souccar's book "Santé, Mensonges et Propagande" (Health, Lies and Propaganda) The book is a real eye-opener and I thoroughly recommend it, if only for the purpose of becoming aware and opening up that space for our own personal choices, which will always be better than some non-independent study.

And this is what we find when we look at what are considered as healthier substitutes.

On one online supermarket that I looked at, this particular snack-bar was classified in the "healthy biscuits" section.

Nutri-Grain Raisin Bakes:

Cereals (36%) (Wheat Flour, Rolled Oats), Glucose-Fructose Syrup, Raisins (10%), Apple Puree, Sugar, Vegetable Oil, Partially Inverted Sugar Syrup, Skimmed Milk Powder, Emulsifiers (E475, E472e, Soy Lecithin), Raising Agent (E500), Flavouring, Modified Starch, Salt, Cinnamon, Barley Malt Extract, Malic Acid, Antioxidant (Ascorbic Acid), Stabiliser (Guar Gum), Niacin, Iron, Vitamin B6, Riboflavin (B2), Thiamin (B1), Folic Acid, Vitamin B12.

The accompanying write-up to the product states that there is nothing "dodgy" in it. Well, for me, E numbers are dodgy, so I find that claim to be rather misleading. Moreover, the product is still processed and contains really a lot of sugar.

I know this may sound that I'm very against sugar and I admit it, I am. Sugar, with today's level of consumption, is a poison. We *can* get away with some, you might not feel so good but your body will be able to deal with it and eliminate it but the trouble is, we are pumping ourselves full of it on a daily basis and, most of the time, without even realizing it. In truth, we are setting ourselves up for some serious health problems at a future point which can be far or frighteningly very near.

Add to that, the large amounts of starch products that we are consuming, for the simple reason that we are told that starch is necessary to fuel our bodies – the GI levels are way above what the human body is programmed and designed to deal with.

Now, don't get me wrong. I'm not saying here that we should never eat bread, rice or pasta. I'm not saying that we should never consume sugar or sugary products. I'm not a no-carbohydrate advocate but I do believe in the way that Nature intended for us and, often, our present way of eating is far removed from Nature.

The Proof of the Pudding is Not in the Added Sugar

We already spoke about how sugar was used for preserving. Salt was also used as a preservative, along with smoking and curing techniques in order to store food.

Previously, the average sugar consumption per person was around a 2lb/1kg bag per year, now we are consuming at least that per person per month, through the sugar that we consume directly and the sugar that is hidden and masked within the foods that we buy.

One of the main advantages of making food from basic ingredients is being able to choose the quantities that you wish to use.

Sugar doesn't really have a taste and when you get used to the taste of more natural, basic foods, anything else, particularly the industrially made foods, just seem very bland.

There's a word in French that I love – "gourmet" I have never been able to find a satisfactory translation in English but the word has it's origin in the French words "gout" meaning taste and "met" meaning the different elements of a meal – a tasty meal with different elements that do not necessarily include the excessive addition of sugar and/or chemical additives.

Sneaky Sweeteners

The major problem with sweeteners is that they fool our bodies into believing that we are eating something sweet when we are not, but they still set off the subsequent mechanisms that are linked to the consumption of sweet foods.

Though they are still largely used, and approved by government bodies, many studies have come out against these sweeteners, particularly aspartame, explaining the grave dangers implied in even a moderate consumption.

The large array of health problems that have their root in the consumption of artificial sweeteners are so many, that it would be easier to discuss the problems they don't cause!

Basically, they cover practically every modern day illness that exists going from the physical – obesity, diabetes, aspartame induced MS, deafness, loss of vision, liver and kidney failure, cancer and neurological disorders – to the psychological – nervosity, irritability, ADD, depression, bipolarity, schizophrenia and suicide. That leaves a rather bitter after taste!

These sweeteners took off in popularity around thirty or so years ago, the marketing pitch told us that their sweetening power was much higher than sugar, thus we didn't need as much, with 0 calories.

My mother was told at the hospital that she wasn't allowed to take sugar, given her diabetic condition, but that sweeteners were perfectly acceptable. My mother was also fairly adept of other sugar-free items – sugar-free chocolate, sugar-free fruit sauce, sugar-free yoghurts, etc – in each product the sugar being replaced by artificial sweeteners.

In later years my mother had enormous problems controlling her diabetes with excessively high and low blood sugars that were largely incomprehensible.

My intuition tells me that all those years of artificial sweetener consumption only went towards largely exacerbating a problem that she may not have experienced without their use.

Of course, it's up to you to decide whether you wish to use sweeteners or not but if you don't wish to, the importance of reading the ingredients on food labels is absolutely essential in order to avoid consuming them unknowingly.

Fast Food Foul-Up – From Opulence to Corpulence

I spent a long time wondering over the reason for existence of fast-food restaurants, which first sprang up in the United States and have now spread almost world wide. (Ironically, we now find certain fast-food restaurants within big cities in countries that are stricken by poverty and famine elsewhere)

Looking back historically, one thing in particular came to my attention which was the American government's desire, at one point, to ensure that all Americans would have enough food to eat and should want for nothing – the idea was to feed every single person in the nation.

This admirable government initiative inspired a lowering of the prices of food but at the same time, there was a progressive lowering of the quality of food. The mass production required preservation techniques in order to transport food over long distances. The industrials had to seek out new methods of preservation and refinement, methods that had to be paid for and then had to become profitable.

Freezers were invented, and then the microwave, the transport system was improved – America was able to hold up to its reputation of being the Land of the Free, where everyone could get a decent bite of the Big Apple.

Unfortunately, the Big Apple had a rather nasty case of worms. The foods that were being made so readily available to the American public were the foods symbolic of opulence, in short, party food - the hamburgers, the fries, the pies, the hotdogs, the doughnuts, the ice-creams, the sodas, to name a few – these were not the foods that comprised the staple of the traditional diet. But now, almost as a show of power, those foods could be bought for next to nothing on the street and in the supermarkets, and were immediately available; somewhere along the line the collective consciousness of the American people was duped into believing that this was good for them.

The fast food market grew and with it the American people's dietary habits took a radical change for the worse, for as the market was growing, at the same time so was the average American's waistline.

We now have a huge problem in the United States some children don't know what vegetables are, who have never seen any. American friends tell me how, in some supermarkets and hypermarkets, there is no vegetable counter and you can't buy anything that hasn't been refined, transformed and had unpronounceable stuff added to it. The restaurants serve up huge amounts of carbohydrate in the form of pizzas, pasta dishes, all high GI and all full of LDL cholesterol.

This problem is no longer contained to the States.

In France, you practically have to bribe the chef in the café-restaurant and canteen to get a bit of green on your plate. The French, who have a long and rich culinary tradition, are losing that identity to the point where, at La Sorbonne university, they have decided to instate a wine tasting moment at lunchtime along with a traditional gourmet meal in the hope of upholding that tradition and identity.

In Britain you now have "all-you-can-eat-buffet" restaurants where for a fixed price you can absolutely stuff yourself silly with food to the point where some restaurant owners have actually banned certain people from coming into their restaurants because, very simply, they eat too much!

A recent documentary by the BBC called "The Men Who Made Us Fat" showed the presenter in a café-restaurant in Brighton that offered three different sizes of English breakfasts. The largest of the breakfasts offered a very generous plate of something in the region of twelve eggs, thirty-six slices of bacon, twenty-four sausages and something in the region of twelve slices of fried bread, a far cry from the more traditional English breakfast which would normally consist of one or two eggs, one or two slices of bacon, one or two sausages, one or two slices of fried bread accompanied by grilled tomatoes and mushrooms. The restaurant owner in this example offered to refund the breakfast to anyone who managed to eat it all – he has had to refund one or two people. The documentary's presenter managed to eat about an eighth of the plate!

The level of excessive gluttony is quite shocking, but the level of waste, when you know that there are people starving elsewhere in the world is, in my humble opinion, very simply abhorrent and more than unnecessary.

✳   ✳   ✳

I would like to discuss, now, some of the foods that are considered or appear natural but that have more or less serious consequences on our health. The first and perhaps the worst of those is milk.

✳   ✳   ✳

Milk Madness

One of the foods that we are told is absolutely necessary for our health and well being is milk. What do we know about it? Milk is full of calcium necessary for the formation and maintenance of bone structure and the prevention of osteoporosis. Milk is full of protein necessary for growth and muscle tonus. Milk is full of fatty acids necessary for the protection against cancer, diabetes and cardio-vascular diseases and help in weight loss and the stabilization of weight. Along with that, we mustn't forget the famous highly beneficial probiotics found in milk that aid our immune system, and lactose lactose, which helps digestion.

Let's have a look at the true and the false in those statements.

Does milk contain a large portion of calcium? Yes, it does. Unfortunately the calcium is not adapted to the human body and is badly assimilated.

Does milk contain large amounts of protein? Yes, it does. Unfortunately, the protein in milk is destined for the consumption of the calf to help the calf grow and is not well adapted for human consumption. Studies over the last thirty years done by researchers from some of the most prestigious universities in the World, including Harvard, have shown that the protein in milk is responsible for the decalcification of bones, obesity, diabetes type I and II and several cancers, not forgetting to mention cardio-vascular diseases.

Some years ago, a colleague of a friend of mine had quite a bad fall while on holiday mountaineering. He broke practically every bone in his body with multiple-fractures and the doctors described his bones as being as brittle as glass. He was in hospital for nearly a year with physiotherapy and re-education that has lasted since. The odd part is, this gentleman in his thirties, who came from the North of France where there is a large dairy tradition, consumed huge amounts of milk and milk products. A bowl of milk in the morning, a yoghurt mid-morning, cheese at every mealtime and a bowl of warm milk before going to bed... With that amount of supposed calcium, it is incomprehensible that his bones should have been so brittle with regards to what we are told about milk.

A contrary example is a neighbour, who also had a very bad fall while out hiking. She broke her leg in one place and was back on her feet as if nothing had happened within six months. My neighbour friend didn't like milk and milk products so never ate them.

Is milk full of beneficial fatty acids? Nope! In a nutshell!

The 'benefits' of the fatty acids in milk, intended for the calf and not for human beings, are largely cancelled out by the excessive amount of proteins.

What of the probiotics? There is absolutely no proof whatsoever that the probiotics in milk protect and aid our immune system. However, several studies have come to light giving evidence that probiotics are responsible for obesity and a whole host of related illnesses. Probiotics were first used for human consumption to combat the effects of anorexia and is widely used to fatten up animals destined for the food market – chickens and pigs primordially.

Does lactose help the digestion of milk? No, it doesn't. In actual fact, human beings are incapable of digesting lactose fairly early in childhood. The reason is very simple. In order to digest the lactose, the body has to produce an enzyme called lactase which breaks down the lactose into two parts that can be assimilated by the human body, galactose and glucose – which is basically sugar but sugar that is designed for small infants and, at that stage, is good for them. Around the age of three to four years old, we stop producing, or we produce only a tiny amount of lactase. The lactose, when consumed at that stage can cause various digestive problems, stomach pains, indigestion, stomach cramps and diarrhoea.

Milk also perturbs the absorption of protective molecules that are present in fruits and vegetables and protect our human cells against old age and illness.

Human beings are the only animals on the planet that continue to consume milk after the period of weaning. My son, around the age of three, just wouldn't eat milk any more, he didn't want it; I would make him a bottle and he would put it in his mouth but not eat it and the bottle would sit there and then I would throw it away. I didn't insist upon him eating it. We are born with a pre-programmed intuition as to what foods are right for us, I felt that if he didn't want it any more then it was because his little body was telling him that he didn't need it any more. Unfortunately, my mother in law who, like many of us, often falls for the media misinformation, in taking care of my son got him back onto drinking milk and for a time, Alistair did consume it again. Now, he very rarely asks for it and I never offer it, but I give him it if he asks; most of the time he doesn't finish it.

Milk production, and all the side-products of milk production, is one of the most lucrative businesses that exist and one of the bases of our modern day economy.

There are many studies claiming the benefits of milk but the milk producers themselves pay for the majority of these studies.

And one important point to bear in mind is the existence of contradictory studies. If milk were in fact good for us, then the entire scientific community would be in agreement on that. The fact that they are not sets off alarm bells for me and brings me back to the same phrase "When in doubt, don't!" – that's my adage, I'm not telling you what to do.

The goal of this is to give you the information that is available so that you can make your own advised choices. Again, once we are aware of the effects, we are in a better position to choose what we want to do.

The Humble Potato

I come from a family where potatoes were a staple in every main meal, cooked in various different forms – boiled, mashed, roasted, baked, chipped and fried, and steamed.
Now, I've had a few friendly "arguments" with people on the subject of potatoes. They are such a common food

item on the plate that for many the idea of only eating them very rarely is quite a strange prospect to them and there is a feeling, at the outset, of something missing.

Contrary to what a lot of people believe, potatoes are not vegetables they are pure starch foods. Now, I like the occasional potato but it's important to know that even in its most basically prepared form it has a really high GI.

To give you an idea, sugar has a GI of 100; a boiled potato has a GI of 85, baked in the oven it has a GI of 95 – it's almost the equivalent of eating pure sugar.

Add to that the tasty toppings of butter, cheese and other delicious ingredients that quite often contain fat, our bodies are in for a lipogenesis party.

Of course, there are contradictory studies that say potatoes are good for us, even a necessary part of our diet, which is interesting because, until the late 1700s, potatoes were not a food that was used for human consumption; they were used however to fatten up the pigs (that was before the invention of probiotics!) and until the late 1700s meat and starch were never mixed together on the same plate. The starch that was eaten mostly consisted of grains and pulses in their brut form, with a very low GI. Most of the time, these grains and pulses would be eaten with vegetables.

Over an eight-month period between 1783 and 1784, the Laki volcano in Iceland entered into eruption blowing poisonous dust and ash high up into the atmosphere. The dust cloud spread across the European continent provoking a momentary but radical climatic change. The dust fell upon fields of crops and entire harvests along with herds of livestock were decimated. It's estimated that this eruption provoked around six million deaths globally and it is suggested to be the root-cause of the French revolution in 1789, due to the extreme poverty and famine that ensued.

In 1785, potato consumption by humans staved off famine in France, largely due to the very clever publicity work of a French chap named Parmentier who, by order of Louis XVI himself, grew potatoes in 15 different plots around Paris, and put his creative skills to inventing as many different recipes as possible with the mature tubers, inviting dignitaries from across the land to try out these new specialities; despite resistance from the Church and the French Medical Faculty.

Parmentier's legacy has left us with the famous French "Hachis Parmentier" (Shepherd's Pie), "Brandade de Morue" (fish pie), the "Gratin Dauphinois," the "Pommes Dauphines," the "Pommes Duchesse," to name a few. It really was a case of making the most of what was available. Once the consumption of those starchy foods had been integrated into the diet, the habit stuck. Potatoes are one of the easiest foods to grow and one of the cheapest to produce and have the added bonus of being filling. With the opening of borders and the improvements in the refinement and transportation systems, pasta and rice were added to the list of starch foods that we now consume on a daily basis; these foods have radically changed, in a very short period of time, what we habitually ate.

Studies in support of the potato and other starch foods, say that they contain a lot of vitamins and vital nutriments that shouldn't be overlooked; some say that potatoes are a rich source of fibre.

First of all, the vitamins and fibre in the potato are contained in and just under the skin, which generally is peeled off; the cooking processes destroy any vitamins that are left and modify the molecular structure turning the potato from a fibrous tuber into a mass of pure carbohydrate. If we were to eat potatoes raw they would have a lower GI and the vitamins may be preserved, but they would be totally inedible, impossible to digest and toxic. Most importantly, the vitamins and fibre, claimed to be found in these foods, can actually be found in higher quantities in foods with a far lower GI.

The other problem with potatoes is that they are really not easily digested, even after the cooking process. Personally, whenever I eat potatoes, I inevitably end up with a bad case of indigestion, which is both unpleasant and embarrassing.

Some people talk about the acid-alkaline incompatibility between starch and protein and there is certainly something in that idea given the digestive reaction that most people experience after eating that particular combination.

The people who have come to me, whom I have assisted in putting into place their own particular natural way of eating, tell me the improvements they experience in the general gastric flow and how much more energy they have. The improvement in digestion is largely due to eating more of the right foods and eating far less foods that are heavy to digest; the improvement in energy levels is simply because the blood sugar levels are behaving within a more normal range, in the way that Nature intended.

Sweetcorn

This is probably the shortest description that I will give in the book. It's called "sweet"corn. The name itself is a giveaway; it has a really high GI. Take into account its transgenic form and it becomes one of the foods that should probably best be avoided!

Again, the argument that the vitamins and nutrients are necessary is a lot of tosh, the same as for potatoes – those vitamins and nutriments can be found in other foods in higher quantities without the glycemic load.

The ancient corn, the corn that the American-Indians ate, didn't present the same problems as our modern day corn but the basic produce has been so transformed by industrial farming that it is a far cry from what it once was.

Add to that, the refining processes – how does a grain of

corn end up being a flake?! – and the addition of sugar to a food that already has a high GI, you get the picture!

Beetroot, Carrots, Turnips and Onions

Everyone has heard of "sugar beet" as a vegetable but it's interesting to note that, particularly here in France, sugar beet is a source of refined sugar production.

It's interesting to note that vegetables that grow underground have a tendency to have a very high GI naturally, including onions. Fry onions until they are light to dark brown, we call that caramelisation, and when cooked they do have a very sweet taste.

However, where I only very rarely eat beetroot, I eat onions fairly regularly. They are not a starch food and as such contain a fair bit of fibre, which lowers the GI. I do think it's best to eat them raw or only very lightly cooked so as not to destroy the cellulose envelope. The grandmother of a friend of mine intuitively claimed that onions were the vegetable of longevity; she lived to the tender age of 95 and in good health too. She also enjoyed garlic on a very regular basis!

Again, as far as beetroot is concerned, though it may have a certain amount of interest from a nutritional point of view; that same interest can be found in other fruits and vegetables without the high GI.

Same for carrots: you can find as much vitamin A in tomatoes as you can find in carrots; and tomatoes, at least the seasonal variety, have been naturally gorged with sunlight – my little finger tells me that's a good thing.

Carrots, when eaten raw, don't have a particularly high GI (of around 30 to 35) however once cooked we're looking at a food that is nearing the sugar equivalent.

Turnips have a similar value, though the assimilation isn't quite the same as is explained in the chapter "The Truth About the Glycemic Index" in part two. Interestingly, certain foods, though containing a high GI don't, however, excessively raise the blood sugar levels.

Coming from Scotland, one of our traditional dishes is "haggis, neeps and tatties" – that would be the famous haggis (ground meat and offal mixed with oats, herbs and spices and boiled in a sheep's stomach), turnip and potatoes. The turnip and potatoes are mashed with lashings of butter – absolutely delicious, but it was not traditionally a feast that people would have other than on a special occasion and nowadays, a lot of Scots don't eat those foods at all. Scotland is yet another country where the culinary tradition has lost a lot of ground, leaving place to some deplorable eating habits, though there is a movement to reinstate traditional cookery, which has a good basis for health.

But again, it's not a question of banishing food but rather being aware of the effects so that we can make advised choices for our diet.

Honey

Honey is a difficult one. It's basically pure sugar, particularly the extract that you find in jars, but does have some very interesting health benefits. Honey can help in boosting your immune system. Add to that the pollen, the royal jelly and the propolys and you've armed yourself with a full natural pharmacy that is very health beneficial.

A while back I watched a series with Jamie Oliver where he visited an apiculture farm and did something that I've always dreamed of doing. He ate the whole honeycomb! It looked amazing!

In the documentary by the Doctor Lustig "Sugar, the Bitter Truth", Dr. Lustig states clearly that nature's kitchen has everything we need as long as we eat the food in its basic natural form. When sugar is present in a fruit or a vegetable, there is always the fibre along with it and the fibre lowers the GI. The problems arise when we extract, transform and refine, only eating the "sweeter" part of the fruit or vegetable. The example given in the documentary was the sugar cane. We eat the sugar but not the cane – if we were capable of eating the woody part along with the sugar it would have far less drastic consequences on our health. Unfortunately, our teeth are not made to be able to deal with that kind of roughage; best leave that kind of work to pandas and such.

Eating honey with the full honeycomb has a similar effect, you get the sugar but the rest of what you are eating largely diminishes the GI.

The Wicked Wheat of the West!

Wheat is everywhere. It's the basis for a good many of the products we buy – bread, pasta, cakes, pastries, cereal bars, pies, tarts, quiches, pizzas, burger rolls, bagels, breaded and battered foods, breakfast cereals. We find extracts of wheat in various forms – wheat syrup to sweeten, wheat gluten and wheat starch to thicken – in foods that have nothing to do with cereal.
One of the main problems with wheat is that invariably we find it in its refined and transformed forms. The refining process, again, removes all the fibre, and thus the nutriments, linked to the basic produce giving it an extremely high GI.
In France, for example, it is unthinkable, for the vast majority of the population, to buy another other type of bread than the white, and very famous, baguette.
My friend's Grandmother, who I mentioned earlier, knew the French bread when it was made with the basic cereal in its natural form; she said that the "traditional" French baguette has absolutely nothing to do with the true "traditional" French baguette. In her days they called it "black bread" and it was made with brut ingredients. It can still be found but only very rarely.

The other major problem with the refined cereal, the refined flour that is used in so many food products, is that it is absolutely loaded with gluten. There is some controversy over whether gluten is "really allergenic" or not but here is what I have learned. The gluten in the bread causes agglutination of blood cells. The white blood cells see this kind of agglutination in the same way as they would see a virus or an infection and thus attack otherwise healthy cells with similar physical reactions in the body as if a true virus or infection were present.

And you don't have to be a celiac sufferer for this to happen. The result is that the body becomes allergic, through the gluten, to other outer elements; so your dust allergy or your cat allergy may just have its origins in gluten intolerance that you're not even aware of.

Wheat has also been show to provoke a demineralization in the body, responsible for bone decalcification – and yet we are told to give milk and bread to our children, supposedly to help them grow and have healthy bones!

However, spelt flour – the ancient, ancient cereal before the Egyptians got their green fingers on it and transformed it into the wheat we know today, does not have the same effect. Though it is still from the wheat family, it does not contain quite the gluten load of our modern day wheat; but is only beneficial to our health as long as we eat the whole spelt and not just the refined part.

Some recent studies of the effects of spelt flour on the GI blood levels, in comparison to those of modern wheat, have stated that there is absolutely no difference. However, it was not specified in the study whether brut or refined cereal were used in the study's investigation.

Other studies on wheat have shown the presence of a chemical substance called acrylamide. This chemical substance, produced when the base ingredient is heated and also found in other cooked starchy foods, has been pinpointed as a carcinogen. Of course, opposing studies are there to say, "No, no, no! – Wheat is good for us!" In France we are told that it an essential part of our diet, especially bread and bread based products.

My own personal experience: I stopped eating modern wheat, apart from the very odd occasion, at the start out when I dropped the 45kg. What was the most notable for me was that up until then I had suffered from tremendous back pains; after about two weeks of having stopped the wheat those pains had totally subsided.
I always choose my foods in their most brut form. For me, eating a grain without the envelope is like receiving a present without the wrapping – missing the essential element!

But once more, this is not a set of rules to follow. I'm aware of the effect wheat has on my body but that doesn't mean that I have totally excluded it from my diet. I don't make life difficult for myself when visiting friends, for example. If I'm presented with foods that are wheat based, I eat them and I enjoy them at the time, I enjoy the social occasion of sharing.

The simple awareness allows me to choose, that is all.

☆   ☆   ☆

I do want to be clear on something here. We've spoken much about the GI levels in food but I am not a low GI proponent as such. I want to be very honest in that I am not a proponent of any kind of diet. The material I studied over the last twenty years or so has brought me to certain conclusions but I feel that as soon as a "label" or a "name" is given to any kind of diet then that diet has a tendency to become restrictive and difficult to maintain, full of rules and regulations that, if not obeyed to the letter, will lead directly to failure and unhappiness.

Yes, I do pay attention to the GI level in the food that I eat but never in an exaggerated manner and I will deal with that in the second part of the book with precise explanations of how the body works but not in order to present you with a set of rules, rather to present you with a true choice.

✳   ✳   ✳

Part 2

In Well-Being, In Well-Eating
The Mind-Body Connection

Obesity is Not a Fatality

*"The greatest fear in the world is of the opinions of others.
And the moment you are unafraid of the crowd you are no
longer a sheep, you become a lion.
A great roar arises in your heart, a roar of freedom"*
Osho

One of the biggest dilemmas that we face when we are overweight, or even if we're not overweight but simply our eating habits are unhealthy, is that we feel stuck in a rut and that it's going to last forever. Add to that the numerous "failed" regimens that we have tried and tested, we end up feeling that we're not getting anywhere, to the point of believing that we can't do it. We are then clouded with thoughts of how unworthy we are as human beings, what losers we are because we seem unable to get ourselves out of this apparently impossible situation. These thoughts can start to affect us in all areas of our lives.

Unfortunately, the media, the marketing professionals and even the medical/nutritional specialists really don't help us in any way to change that image we have of ourselves.
We are told that we have slow metabolisms, that we have medical conditions or medical history that won't allow us to improve our health. The media and marketing professionals use the weakness of our seemingly desperate situation to attempt to sell us the magic solution – pills, potions and powders that come accompanied by marvellous claims of how they will improve our weight and our health – but that ultimately will not make the slightest bit of difference. We automatically assume that it is our fault and that we're the ones not making enough effort. The idea that these miracle solutions don't actually work doesn't seem to enter into our thinking.

We are continually beating ourselves up, creating a vicious circle where, indeed, we feel there is no way out. We look in the mirror and are unhappy with what we see, we double up on our determination and decide at those moments that we should or shouldn't eat this or that – except of course we're going to be invited out for tea or dinner or something will happen and we'll eat a food that isn't in our new prescribed set of rules and that's it, we're back to square one – losers, unworthy human beings, ugly and trapped! We heave a huge sigh of self-disappointment, go to sleep, get up the next day, look in the mirror and the whole cycle starts all over again.

One of my friends recounted her story of when she was on the Mayo diet. She had started on the Monday and was doing really well "sticking to it" but then came Sunday and Sunday she went to church where communion was held. Being quite devout, she took communion and then felt terrible because she had a tiny sip of wine and a morsel of bread, feeling that she had just ruined her diet and all the efforts that she had been making.

I would like to think of this as an exceptional example but we see this around us every day – people on more or less restrictive diets, making these superhuman efforts to stay on them and feeling awful about themselves if they make the tiniest divergence. Moreover, witnessing that and realizing that we do these restrictive diets, fully believing that they're healthy, while completely ignoring how we are feeling physically and psychologically.

We see it all the time; the young woman, desperate to lose weight, on a madly restrictive diet, undergoing symptoms of fatigue, hunger, hypoglycaemia, frustration, irritability, depression but somehow, in the collective mind, this is good for us?

These reactions are the signal that we're not doing what our bodies need but instead of tuning into that and responding to those needs, we "step up" in motivation and go and do two hours worth of exercise, ultimately heightening the symptoms. Sure the endorphin release will give the impression that everything is as it should be but that "good" feeling is ephemeral and once the endorphin levels diminish, the sensations of fatigue, hunger, hypoglycaemia, frustration, irritability and depression, return with fervour.

If you were sent to a labour camp where you were required to exercise while being subjected to food deprivation, you would be suffering and searching for a means of escape, yet there are men and women throughout our Western civilisation who subject themselves freely and deliberately to that kind of treatment on a daily basis. How can we possibly believe that that is good for us?

We are constantly taught in our society that self-criticism will be a motivating factor in getting us into gear and that if we are not getting the results we alone are responsible; we are lazy, not committed enough, lacking willpower, weak. Although those are nothing more than misplaced accusations, we believe them to be true and so pursue in our superhuman efforts to try and resolve what we believe is an enormous problem, and what we are told is an enormous problem.

I have never yet met one person with a weight challenge who has not wanted their body to be different and who was not, at least 90% of the time, making huge efforts to do something about their condition.
The constant bombardment of super healthy images – lean, muscular and extremely handsome young men; slender, graceful and beautiful young women - the one thing these images all have in common, other than the airbrushing, is that they make us feel crap and most of

the time it is done deliberately in order to sell us something. The media projected image is telling us that our own personal projected image is ugly, but buy the product and you're going to feel and look like Mr. or Mrs. Gorgeous!

I ended up never looking at myself in the mirror and I know that from having spoken with others that I'm not alone in this. The reflected image didn't fit in with society's requirements, I felt extremely ugly.

But who says that you're not beautiful or handsome? The truth is, it's yourself who is saying that, if you're feeling that way it's because you, yourself, are thinking it.
You see, if it was just society on the outside saying it then it would just be society on the outside saying it. But when we take it on board, when we think it ourselves, and goodness knows everything is designed for us to do so, and if we believe what we are thinking then we feel we are ugly, unworthy losers. And how in the heck are we supposed to take care of ourselves and be nice to ourselves when we have such low opinions of ourselves? If a friend or spouse were to call you to your face the above names or similar, would you feel like being nice to them?
And yet, that is what we do to ourselves, every single day. We insult ourselves and then put ourselves through torture, punishing ourselves through deprivation and frustration, in the hope that we will lose those extra pounds and finally be allowed to be happy, just like the adverts!

You Don't Have to Weight to Be Happy!

When you are in a different mindset weight loss is completely without effort at all – my goal is to help you get to a place where, as I did, you can and will do it without even having to think about it. And the really good news is that, once you have the understanding of where all of that is coming from, it's as simple as saying, *"hello."*

One of the exercises I do with my clients is to get them to look in the mirror, just at their face and to make a mental, or written if they wish, note of what is beautiful. I bet you've got gorgeous eyes! How about a flash of that stunning smile? Maybe you've got a sweet little button nose (I hope so – mine is a little sharp and pointy but it's still my nose and I can still breathe through it)

But the most essential part of the work I do is helping people to realize that the outer carapace is not who they are. Inside of that carapace, whatever its shape or size, resides a beautiful soul, a miraculous, unique and marvellous gift to this earth. The love in your heart is who you are. How you treat other people with kindness is who you are. Your sense of humour is who you are. Your intelligence and, above all, your wisdom is who you are. Your soul essence is who you are. The outer shell is what all of that lives and breathes in. The physical appearance of the outer shell doesn't really have that much importance.

The only thing I'm concerned with, regarding your outer shell, is how it affects your health, general vitality and internal body chemistry. For me, a weight problem is not a problem, it's just something to be gently dealt with and then released.

Ask yourself these questions: If you weren't reliant on losing weight in order to feel happy and good about yourself, how would you eat differently? How would you feel differently about having that cake when invited to dinner? How would your ideas and feelings around food be different? How would it be if you could take away the importance of what food means to you? How would it make you feel right now to take that pressure off?

Obesity is not a fatality, not even for those with a medical condition. When you tap into your intuition that will tell you the foods that you need and you become aware of and listen to your body, you will be naturally attracted to different foods than those that you have perhaps felt compelled to eat in the past.

The Difference Between Food-Wants and Food-Needs

One evening, on a conference coaching call with Michael Neill, one of the subjects being discussed was the difference between "wants" and "needs". Now, Michael explained this difference as, and this is really just common sense, a "want" being something that you would like but has no particular consequence if you don't have it and a "need" being something that is necessary to do or have lest there be some kind of consequence. For example a "want" would be living in that amazing house on the edge of a lake, but if I don't I'm not any the less happy for it, and a "need" would be making sure I pay my electricity bill or I run the risk of having the electric company cut the power.

You could define a want as something internal to yourself that can bring you some kind of pleasure, and a need as an external element needing to be dealt with.

There are many elements in life that could enter into both of those categories as a want and a need; food is one of them.

We need to eat food for our health, to maintain our cellular structure and body functions. We want food because it tastes nice and it's pleasurable.

Now, the difficulty that a lot of us have is combining the food "need" and the food "want" in a manner that is both healthy and enjoyable. We associate certain meanings to different foods. For a very long time sweets were symbolic to me of a treat or a special occasion, boiled eggs were symbolic of my Grandparents and the associated happy memories, cabbage and gravy were symbolic of warmth during winter. There's nothing particularly wrong with associating some kind of symbolic to foods, the key is realizing that you're the one deciding on that symbolic, you're the one thinking about it in that way, you're the one giving the importance or not to those foods. We have to admit that there is a fair bit of psychology going on behind the way we eat.

A shift in the connection that we have towards food goes a long way in helping us make the right choices and being happy about them. Having the knowledge of how our bodies work and the effect that foods have on our systems, albeit positive or negative, combined with this shift in the mindset is really the key to obtaining the results that you would like to see.

When you're in a high state of mind, feeling happy and at peace within yourself, you don't have to push yourself to make any particular food choices, it just happens naturally. You automatically feel like taking care of yourself and you don't question it or think about it.

On the other hand, when you are in a low state of mind, feeling down, it can be incredibly hard to make yourself eat healthier foods or even simply to be kind to yourself. It's all very well to say, *"don't eat less, do eat better"* but unless you have the keys in hand to be able to do that, it's not going to serve any long-lasting purpose.

One of those keys is being kind to yourself, giving yourself a break. You're a wonderful human being. I see the light in you. What will make this easy is seeing that light in yourself, becoming aware of it.

The Problem with Motivation and Willpower

For me, there is a huge problem with the ideas of motivation and willpower.

Each of these words automatically requires that we search for some reason or element outside of ourselves in order to do something; in our case, to lose weight and be healthier. A lot of the time, that outside reason or element is the wanting to be accepted by society, to fit in. But in reality, it doesn't matter how thin you are – thinness doesn't bring happiness, thinness doesn't bring love and thinness doesn't bring wealth and riches. Being thin doesn't bring us more friends, doesn't make us more or less acceptable by society; but it's what we think, it's what we believe. If you imagine that you're not acceptable, you're not going to go out towards others and when we're overweight, we tend to believe that we are less acceptable than others and more likely to be judged.

The truth is, whatever your physical appearance happens to be, we are all judged and we all judge on all sorts of different aspects, not just physical appearance. We judge whether someone is nice or not, we judge according to our own belief systems and education. The key of the "how to" not let that get to us is very simple. Judgement is nothing more than a person's personal thought and only has the importance that they, or we, give to it, but it's not because somebody else thinks something that it is either true or that we have to think it too.

One of the most insightful experiences I ever had was watching a group of people walking down the road, each of them thinking, it was visible by their facial expressions. Everybody thinks, that's common knowledge; what seems to be less apparent is that each and every one of us is creating a reality through our own thinking, a perception of our surroundings that is nothing more than illusion.

If you can imagine a group of people in space suits with those spherical space helmets; they are in their own personal little bubble with their thinking, with the ability to communicate outside of themselves, and each with their own perception of what they see on the outside. We use our thinking to navigate through our surroundings, it's a tool, but that doesn't mean that what we think is necessarily true. When we can waken up to the illusion of our own thinking, when we see that we are literally making it up as we go along, it becomes clear that neither our own personal judgement of a person or circumstance, nor another person's judgement of us has any importance at all. We can change our minds at any moment on any subject; how many times has it happened that we've misjudged a person to then decide that this person wasn't as bad as we thought, or is even pretty nice. None of what we think is real, all we have done is change our minds, change our thinking.

When you can see that a person who misjudges you is only doing it because they believe that their own thinking is real, then you don't have to give any importance to that person's thoughts. Until somebody taps us on the shoulder and awakens us to the illusion of thought, we believe, in all innocence, that we are right and justified in the thinking that we have; we will even back it up from past experience but that too, is nothing more than supplementary thought.

One of the most fundamental things that I've noticed is that, when you're not taking another person's thinking seriously, because you are aware that it's just their thinking, oddly enough that person will very naturally change their mind without you having to do or say anything – you just have to be your beautiful self. You will see that, no matter what your physical appearance may be, people will warm to you and be naturally drawn to you; when we see all thought as illusion we lose our own sense of righteous judgement on others and we very naturally touch a wealth of compassion; people are drawn to that.

Ultimately, the only barrier to your own happiness, health and friendship with others, is thought and let's face it, it's not as if we can hold a thought in our hands.

> *Because one believes in oneself, one doesn't try to convince others. Because one is content with oneself, one doesn't need others' approval. Because one accepts oneself, the whole world accepts him or her ~ Lao Tzu*

The only thing that being slimmer or thinner can bring you is health, that's the only thing. And the only thing health will do is make your life physically easier.

It all comes down to the same thing – we are continually looking on the outside for things that will make us happy on the inside. But here's the beautiful part, we don't need anything on the outside to make us happy on the inside because being happy on the inside is already there. The only thing that stops us feeling happy in the moment is our own thinking; inner happiness, inner well being is just one thought away.

At the outset, when I started losing weight, I did it without even realizing it. I had actually given up the idea of ever losing weight. I had tried so many different diets and concoctions in order to reach the societal "ideal weight" that it had just got too much. I was in constant emotional pain until one morning I got up, struggled to get myself straightened up, and without realizing, decided that was it – I wasn't even going to try any more, I was in a place of acceptance. It was already a struggle physically, I didn't want to struggle psychologically any more.

But being in a place of acceptance doesn't mean to be in a place of lassitude. This is where we tend to go wrong. We believe that if we let go of the control of what we're eating, then we will either not do anything about it at all or we will eat even worse.

That's not what acceptance is about. This is acceptance of the idea that we are the ones making up all the really hard rules to follow, that we're the ones giving the importance to the foods that we eat, we're the ones deciding that it's bad to eat this and good to eat that and that if we don't comply with our made-up rules then we are bad people. When we accept that we're the ones doing it to ourselves, miraculously, and I say that with no exaggeration, all of those extraneous unhelpful thoughts just melt away. What we are left with is Wisdom and Intuition; we are left with a quieter mind, which allows us to tune into our bodies and listen for what we need. In the same way as a radio signal can be disrupted by other signals, satellite dishes, you name it, leaving us unable to hear what's being said; when we switch off all of those external elements, the white noise disappears and what we're left with is a pure signal with no disturbance that we can hear perfectly.

Accepting that we are the ones doing the thinking and creating our own reality, literally creating moment to moment our experience of life, is the way to get onto the clear channel where there is no doubt about the intuitive messages that are being given.

But the choice is there, we can choose to continue to make up tons of rules about what we should or should not be eating, leading our lives in an atmosphere of "motivation" and "will-power," which is ultimately a lot of hard work through self-created suffering, or we can let go and ease ourselves onto that Gentle Path that will in due course lead us to Definitive Weight Loss.

I knew, through all the literature that I'd been reading over all those years, what to eat so that I would at least be healthy on the inside and so I started doing that and it was made all the more easy that I had completely taken the pressure off.

I'm not saying that I wanted to remain at the weight that I was carrying at that time but what is for sure is that I wasn't making myself any more unhappy by putting myself through the treadmill in order to achieve some far away goal that I wasn't even sure I could attain.

And so what happened was, in a healthy optic, I just put into place what I knew using the food that I like to eat. For example, I love chocolate and so when I wanted something sweet I would go into the cupboard. At first my hand would automatically reach for the packet of biscuits but I would still myself, move my hand to the left and take the bar of dark chocolate that was sitting next to them instead. Because I didn't have the pressure of "having to not eat" the biscuits, there wasn't any problem in taking something else that I liked instead – I wasn't having the dark chocolate in order to lose weight, I was having the dark chocolate because I liked it.

I was discussing with a client one evening who was beating himself up quite a lot for his "bad eating habits" and for "allowing himself to fall into temptation with that cake." The penny dropped for him when I pointed out that if he were in perfect health, if he didn't feel that there was something wrong with him, if he didn't feel that he was unacceptable by society, he would just have eaten the cake without batting an eyelid; after all I've never heard a "healthy, thin person" have a go at themselves because they had a cake. If your response to that is, "Yes, but they're healthy and thin, they can 'afford' to have the cake," be aware that you just made up a new rule about yourself.

And so it was for the rest of my eating habits. Because I wasn't making an effort to lose weight, I wasn't holding that as an objective any more, then there was no pressure for me to do anything – I was free to choose.

About one month after having 'given up,' I was putting on my bra and couldn't do it up. I thought it was broken and took it off several times to look at it but the catches were all intact and in the right places so I couldn't understand what was happening until I suddenly realized that when I pulled the bra round, the clasps were no longer aligned. And that's when I suddenly noticed that all of my clothes were looser on me – I was stunned.

Then the motivation came back. Seeing that I was getting a result by not making any effort whatsoever, just by doing things very simply and eating food that I like, gave me the will to carry on not making any effort. I was enjoying the food that I was eating, and still do, and at the same time, I could see and feel differences in my body and was enjoying that too. But I didn't make it happen, I allowed it to happen.

There's another important thing to bear in mind with regards to motivation and willpower and our belief that happiness will come when we achieve what we believe we desire.
Human beings adapt, we get used to living in a certain way; we are creatures of habit. It is our capacity for adaptation that has helped us survive through the ages, through difficult times and also through good times.

When we are overweight, we adapt to that situation too. The first time someone calls us a fat slob is far more hurtful than the 100th or the millionth time someone calls us a fat slob – I'm not saying that it's nice but we still do adapt.
Of course you will feel a certain amount of satisfaction and pleasure when you lose weight, I know I did, but satisfaction and pleasure are not long-term emotional states. We adapt to our environment, we adapt to the

new weight that we are now living with – you will get used to it, so that new weight that you believed would make you happy will ultimately just become everyday and normal. The thrill will dissipate.

That's not to belittle the achievement, it's a fantastic achievement, but to point out that long-term happiness doesn't come from that. Your sense of happiness, peace and well being is accessible to you at any moment, the only barrier to that is your own thinking.

I've been living now for around five years in what can be called a normal sized body, I'm used to it now. I'm glad of it but my sense of inner well being is not affected by whatever weight I happen to be. That also makes things easier when I put on a little bit during the holiday seasons – it takes away all the drama. So, I put on a little during those periods because I'm eating foods that are exceptional but I don't panic or worry about it. I know that I'll come back to my usual way of eating and that the weight will drop again – it doesn't become a big deal.

Thus it is in this built-in capacity for adaptation that resides our most beautiful and precious power: our power of inner well being. Human beings adapt and become accustomed to any situation, the only thing that stops us feeling happy in the moment is our own thinking, our own thoughts. Why is it that one person suffering from an illness just gets on with life, managing his or her condition as if nothing was amiss whereas another person stops living completely, becomes embittered with life and feels that without that illness they could have been so much happier and done so many things? Why is one person happy while the other is a victim?
The only difference is Thought!

One last word on *motivation* and *will power.* The word *motivation* comes from the Latin word *movere*, which simply means *to move*. The psychological use of the word *motivation* to mean *"inner or social stimulus for an action"* only came into being in 1904! Up until then, it just meant *motion*. Another way of saying that would be, **"being in the flow."**

Will power is simply the power of wanting. We spoke earlier about a "want" being something that would bring us enjoyment, so will power is, in the end, simply the **"power of enjoyment"**

The Power of Innate Well Being

"Thought is a divine tool, nothing more, nothing less, only a tool.
A wise person, like a good tradesman, uses this tool to the best of his or her ability"
Sydney Banks

As human beings we have three very basic needs for our physical and emotional well being: eating, drinking and sleeping. We can include other needs such as warmth and friendship but if the first three are covered, then we have all we need. It is undeniable that eating properly, drinking fresh water and sleeping enough hours play an important role in our well being. Those three elements greatly affect our body chemistry. If you don't get enough sleep; you are going to feel tired and grumpy, lethargic, perhaps even a little sad or depressed. Lack of sleep affects the brain chemistry. Eat unhealthily and the brain chemistry will be affected in the same way.

If I am, personally, eating a diet that has too high a GI, I find myself more inclined to have negative thoughts and, more importantly, to give importance to those negative thoughts. But the beautiful part is this: as human beings we have the free will to choose which thoughts to give power to. It is our thinking that creates our reality, our perception of what is going on around us - this is why you have people who can be living in the most abject poverty but who are still happy within themselves and others who can have everything that a person could ever want materially but who are deeply and profoundly unhappy.

As children, we take things in our stride - circumstances can change but we adapt and continue to live in that sense innate happiness and well being within ourselves. Notice when a child gets upset. Oftentimes he or she may just be tired or hungry. What's important to notice is that one second a child may be in tears and the next laughing his or her head off. A child has not gained the learned ability of fixing him or herself onto any particular thought - a child allows the thoughts to pass, fresh thinking is just around the corner.

We are, indeed, just one thought away from true happiness.

As adults, we learn the "pursuit of happiness." We need "success" - but what is a successful life? Is it the balance in your bank account? The car you drive? The holidays you go on? The house you live in? The way you look and dress?
These are only outer exhibits of financial/material gain and in no way are a guarantee of a person's happiness; they also don't mean anything about the person. Take it all away and the person, in essence, is still the same. True success is living in a feeling of innate well being, knowing that no matter what happens on the outside, we all have the ability to tap into our inner resources of resilience, peace and wisdom.

There is a world of difference between happiness and pleasure/enjoyment. Having the car you want may bring you pleasure but will never give you that long lasting sense of well being. Pleasure and enjoyment can only ever be temporary; again you will get used to driving that car, it may break down and then you may even feel a sense of annoyance, anger, and deception.

What I want to show you is that steadfast and unshakeable sense of well being that no amount of material gain can bring you and that no one can take away from you.

When you know within yourself that your rock solid well being is not dependant on having all the material things, and never has been, you open a door to endless possibility.

At one point in my life I went through a phase of not seeing the point of doing anything, not because I was afraid of anything but simply because I was feeling so well in myself that I didn't feel the need to do anything - I didn't need anything to feel happy, happiness was already there just as it is already there in each and every one of us. The insight I had was realizing that I can do things simply because I enjoy them. Writing a book is pleasurable, talking with people is pleasurable, going for a walk on a beach is pleasurable, driving in the countryside is pleasurable but without those extra things, I would still feel very happy and at peace.

When you know within yourself the difference between happiness and enjoyment, not only do you gain an enormous amount of resilience but you also open the door to trying anything you would like to do. Because your own happiness is not dependant on "such-and-such" coming to fruition, you then simply have the enjoyment of making a go of it and if it doesn't work out, it doesn't matter. You are independent of the result.

But I will say this... For all those things that you would like to do or obtain - having a sense of inner well-being and peace will allow you to tap into that source of inner wisdom that we all have and you won't even need to make the effort to "make things happen" - they will happen all by themselves....

And the same is true around the subject of weight loss and health. When you are in that place where you are no longer reliant on the result for your happiness and are already in your state of inner well-being, as I did, you will lose weight without the trouble and strife, and, most likely, without even realizing it... *The power of enjoyment in the flow*

The Stress Factor

"You cannot be made to feel anything you cannot think"
Keith Blevens

A recent documentary series by the Dr. Robert Lustig and his team, who I admire for their great work, mentioned, in one of the episodes, the stress factor.
There have been medical studies concerning the effects of stress on weight gain. One study, documented in the series "The Skinny on Obesity" by Dr Robert Lustig and carried out in a sample group of around fifty women, concluded that stress did indeed cause an increase in fat around the stomach, hips and thighs. These studies are based on a fundamental misunderstanding of the nature and role of stress in our lives.

So let's take a look at where stress comes from. Imagine the following: you're sitting in the library writing an essay that is due for the next day. The person at the next table is sitting with a newspaper and babbling away on their mobile phone. In the paradigm that we are taught, this person is causing you stress – they are disturbing and distracting you, preventing you from concentrating and getting on with the really important work that you have to do.
Here is the reality of the situation:
The person is using a mobile phone in a place where it's not allowed.
The person is making some noise and disturbing the people around them, which is why mobile phones in

libraries are not allowed.

The stress that you are feeling is not however coming from that person; the stress is actually coming from your own thinking. You start the process by thinking something along the lines of: "this person is really rude:" "I can't concentrate because of the noise:" "I'm not going to get my work finished in time:" "why can't they just bugger off and have their big long mobile phone conversation in a more suitable place, like a café?"

The phenomena is then exacerbated by the fact that the mobile phone conversation continues and you have the same thoughts repeating themselves in your mind, increasing the feelings of stress and fear that you're not going to get your work finished on time. Now, you are not only distracted by the person on the phone, you are also greatly distracted by your own thoughts. The fact is that most of the time we are unaware that it is our own thinking that creates the feelings of stress/fear/anger and not the outside element. Now, I'm not saying that it's not annoying to have a situation like that to deal with but our stressful thoughts around that situation exacerbate what is really happening.

Everything we feel in the moment is directly linked to what we are thinking in the moment. We have between something like 70 000 to 120 000 thoughts per day. A single thought can instantaneously make us feel stressed/fearful/angry or happy/content/at ease. And as Dr. Bill Pettit, psychiatrist, points out, having stressful thoughts over as short a time as 3 to 5 minutes is enough to modify the brain chemistry, pulling us into a low state of mind.
What's important to know is that a thought is completely neutral: it's nothing more than an electrical impulse designed to help us navigate our surroundings. As human beings, we have the capacity to put words onto those electrical impulses and give them a meaning

that is either positive or negative.

Recognizing that stressful thoughts come from within and not from what is happening on the outside is the key to dealing with whatever life presents to us. They always say, "in case of fire, stay calm" – the reason for that is simple, when in a calm state we have more chance of escaping unharmed, simply because we are thinking clearly.

So in our library example we have several possibilities: we can get ourselves completely wound up, leave the library with a sense of disgust, stress and anger and go buy a cream cake, or we can recognize that the stress is coming from our own thinking and politely ask the person to take the phone call outside; move to another area of the library; inform a librarian and ask them to intervene; in a higher state of mind, when our thoughts aren't racing, there is a whole host of calm solutions that we can come up with in the face of such a problem.

This is what I felt was missing with the study done by Dr. Lustig and his team, in all innocence. It is simply not in our classical school education to realize that our own thinking creates our reality. We all have different techniques for stress management, which ranges from breathing deeply and counting to ten before "reacting", to taking pills and making regular visits to a psychiatrist. Many of those techniques will work in the moment but they have to be done over and over again, this is why it is called "stress management" not "stress healing". When we realize that everything we are feeling and experiencing as reality is coming from within ourselves via thought, then the simple act of recognizing that is the catalyst for letting go – so no need for cream cakes as a stress-relief but they are still perfect for parties and pleasure.

The Great Thought Illusion

The truth is, we are the creators of our own experience of life; that is to say that whatever we think we feel. If you have angry thoughts, you will feel angry, if you have loving thoughts, you will feel loving. Conversely, you cannot have a loving thought and feel angry and vice versa. This much every single human being on Earth can understand.

What we can have more difficulty understanding, though it is so beautiful in its simplicity, is that we are, in fact, the ones doing the thinking.

So what is a thought? Since the beginning of the time of man, thought, whether verbalized or not, is the tool that we use to navigate our environment in much the same way as every living creature on Earth uses thought. Thought, as an electro-neural impulse, is what helps us get out of danger, allows us to find food – it is a tool for survival.

In the case of Homo sapiens, it's an ultra-developed navigation system that we have verbalized and intellectualized. Strangely enough, the term Homo sapiens means "wise man", yet we can appear to be anything but wise, particularly in committing acts of violence and destruction.

So why is that? Well, it's fairly simple to understand. When we take our own thoughts very seriously and believe what we are thinking, we feel that we don't have any choice but to act upon our thoughts. We believe so ardently in the righteousness of our own thinking, we are blinded to the fact that there can be any other possible way of "navigating the surroundings".

You see - thought is an illusion. If you take two different people and put them in exactly the same set of circumstances, one may find those circumstances unbearable while the other finds them perfectly acceptable or even pretty cool!

When we look on situations of that kind, we will say that one is weak and one is strong and brave and positive but that's not it. As human beings we are all made equal; what differentiates us is the way we think about things. The one who finds the circumstances horrible finds it so because of their thoughts, the one who finds the same circumstances acceptable or even pleasant, finds it so because of their thoughts.

Our thoughts create our feelings and we are the ones doing the thinking.

But there is no obligation to think whatever we may be thinking, we can think something completely different but we get stuck in our thinking and can't see any other way out than the way we are choosing to navigate.

What makes the difference in the way we choose to navigate is WISDOM.

Unfortunately we can get caught up with the same thoughts turning round and round in our brains, unable to let go of them... in all innocence.

And I say "in all innocence" because we are brought up to believe that it is our outside circumstances that dictate how we feel and we are jumping a step; that step is thought. The link between our circumstances and our sentiment of those circumstances is thought.

If person A believes that person B is responsible for their anger, hurt, negativity, even circumstances, then person A is likely to take their anger out on person B.

But if person A is aware of the fact that they are creating their own experience of life, and that they have no obligation to think what they are thinking, then they become fully responsible of their own thoughts and thus, their own acts.

Thought is like an optical illusion; until we see the illusion we believe it's real – we see the face of an old lady when we could be seeing the face of a young woman because this much is true: we see what we choose to see, the importance is realizing that we have a choice.

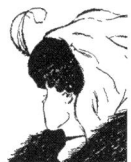

The difference between the "outside in" and the "inside out" paradigm: The first are living in an illusion and seeing it as reality, the second are living in a reality and seeing it as illusion.

'People Labels' and How to Rid Them

"There are only two kinds of eaters; the Anteater and the Beefeater"
Unknown

There are number of labels that we use, consciously and unconsciously, to justify our eating habits. I carry no judgement in those words, as I too, carried a label and justified my eating habits with them for a very long time.

Ever since human beings developed the ability to articulate words and give names to things, we have, through time, developed the habit of giving names to, and categorizing, everything and everyone around us. We categorize others by: country, "race", colour, gender, gender preference, age, abilities, good or bad. We then add to that a whole number of sub-categories: helpful - unhelpful, selfish - generous, rich - poor, pretty - ugly, phoney - natural, co-dependent - independent... the list goes on and on.

Thus our ability to use a word to describe an object has become a tool of judgement towards others and ourselves.

When it comes to the labels that we give ourselves concerning our eating habits, the list again is long. We have the emotional/comfort eater, heredity, big-boned, defeatist, unworthy/unloved, can't be done, big eater, bulimic, anorexic, etc.

The one thing that all of the labels that we use have in common is that they present a catch 22 situation – they are, each and every one of them, a trap... but a homemade trap.

I remember one day having a discussion with my mother. I had put on a fair bit of weight at the time and my mother said to me that she had always found that I was a bit of a comfort eater. She wasn't saying that to be horrible, on the contrary she was quite concerned to see that I had put on so much weight in such a short space of time. Before that conversation I had never thought of myself as a "comfort eater", but once she said it I started thinking, "oh yes, she's right. I am a comfort eater. When things go 'wrong' I automatically eat a whole lot of food that is fattening" and so I started consciously wearing that label.

The problem of course is that with the label, I felt didn't have a choice. Labels are anchored in the collective mind and, with the risk of repeating myself too often, the media do everything they can to maintain those labels. Just, for a moment, imagine what it would be like if you didn't wear that label any more. Imagine how freeing that would be. Imagine what you would be able to choose to do or not to do.

Take any of the above labels and you have the following vicious and painful cycle:
You are in a situation of unhealthy eating habits – you

make an effort to improve those eating habits – you create for yourself feelings of frustration/privation/guilt – you remind yourself that you are "...insert label..." – you "punish yourself" by "giving in" to what you believe you should not be doing – you then beat yourself up for having done that... and so on and so forth... and round and round we go...

We are the only species on Earth that develop bad eating habits, restrain ourselves, punish ourselves and worry about all of that. We are also the only species on Earth that can express thought through words.

When we recognize the nature of thought, and the power that it holds over us if we are not aware that we are the thinker, then we are able to let go of all of those labels. We realize that we are doing it to ourselves and we don't have to, making it very easy to tune into nature as we have been created to do and tune into our natural intuition around our eating habits, which will let us know unambiguously what is right for us and what is not right for us.

There is a wonderful simplicity of recognizing thought - when we say to ourselves "bollocks! I've had a really bad day, it's been really stressful, I had to deal with all of those horrid people, etc, etc, I'm going to have a bigmac/cream cake/mars bar/pork pie to make myself feel better", we can recognise that all of that is just thought, including the stressful thoughts that we may have had throughout the day. This gives us the key to not having those thoughts take over and rule our lives, our actions or reactions and our eating. We can still choose to go and have that bigmac/cream cake/mars bar/pork pie but we know then that it's our own choice and that we're not being pushed to do it by an outer force going against our will.

The simple fact of recognizing that we are the thinker

allows the thoughts to slow down. When our thinking slows down, fresh new thinking can spring up. This fresh thought can take the form of calm ideas and gentle solutions that enable us to work through the things we have to deal, without making ourselves unhappy and without having to rely on an "eating mechanism" for our well-being.

Our well being is already within us and the only thing that stops us tapping into it and thriving is our own thinking.

We Are the Universe

"Do you not know that you are God's temple and that God's Spirit dwells in you?"
Bible

"When he turns his back, his aim everywhere is to spread mischief through the earth and destroy crops and cattle. But Allah loveth not mischief"
Qur'an

We are part of Nature, we are made from the creative energy of the universe and, as such, are inseparable from it but human beings, unlike any other species on Earth, have developed a way of living that goes against Nature and Universal Laws. The only explanation of this fact is that we have learned over time that well being comes from the outside of us and not from within. Our ego develops from this and from ego comes greed and materialism. Our world is full of people obsessed with financial profit who, despite their inner knowing, will do whatever they consider necessary to make that profit, no matter what the human and environmental cost. It comes down to a question of control. Some people believe that by controlling everything outside of themselves, no matter what that implies for the planet, then they will be happy. I have yet to meet one of those people who were not fooling themselves and who deep down didn't know that. We can't either control the thoughts that pop up in our heads, however we can control the importance and the focus that we give to those thoughts – the only power we really have, and it is a marvellous blessing, is the power of free-will with the capacity to choose which thoughts to give our attention to.

This paradigm that we are living, where we seek happiness on the outside of ourselves is recent. Take any ancient writing and you quickly discover that we have always known that we are a part of the Universe and that the Universe resides within us – every single religion, every single spiritual teaching on Earth carries that basic message.

One of my favourite quotes is from the astrophysicist Neill de Grasse-Tyson, which beautifully sums up our connection to Nature and the Universe:

> "The most astounding fact... is the knowledge that the atoms that comprise life on Earth, the atoms that make up the human body are traceable to the crucible, (of creation) of all the fundamental ingredients of life itself...
>
> ... When I look up at the night sky, I know that we are part of the Universe, we are in this Universe but, perhaps more important than both of those facts, is that the Universe is in us.
> When I look up and reflect on that fact, I feel big because my atoms come from these stars.
> There's a level of connectivity... That's really what you want in life, you want to feel connected, you want to feel relevant, you want to feel participant in the goings-on of activities and events around you.
> That's precisely what we are... just by being alive..."

The next time you are in a forest, remember that you are part of that forest. The next time you are by the ocean, remember that the ocean is within you. The next time you look up at the night sky and contemplate the moon and the stars, remember that you are the moon and the stars, remember that you are made up of exactly the same stuff.

We are of this Universe as is every living plant, tree and animal on this planet. We are all made of the same molecules and particles. Our contra natural way of living is destroying us and destroying this miraculous planet that we live on. By disrespecting Nature, we thus disrespect ourselves. One thing that I always keep in mind when I am eating is that I am replenishing my body with the energy of life itself. When that energy has been modified and transformed into something other than what it was intended to be, I can only deduce that that modification and transformation will show up, in one way or another, within my body.

In Nature, by eating basically and naturally, we can find absolutely everything we need to live a healthy, full and happy life. Each and every natural whole food found in Nature holds all the bits and pieces of atoms and molecules that we need to replenish our bodies and, as if that wasn't miraculous enough, in those foods can be found cures for illnesses. There are foods out there that will help you produce interleukin 2, a molecule used in chemotherapy, very naturally with no adverse side effects. There are foods that produce powerful antibacterial and antiviral effects. There are foods for replenishing the cells in our bodies, foods that keep our bodies healthy and young, foods that get rid of free radicals, others that act as antioxidants.

The truth of the Miracle is that we have all the resources that we need, right there within Nature, literally at our fingertips, and presented to us on a beautiful planet that we have named Earth. So it becomes completely incomprehensible that we fill ourselves full of food that has been so transformed and modified that it has the exact opposite effect on our body than Nature intended.

Just to be clear once more – I'm not some goody two shoes that never eats a doughnut, or an ice cream – of course I do but I don't make a daily habit out of it but most of all, I don't make a big deal out of it when I do.

Preconceived Ideas

There are a number of preconceived ideas that are bandied about, usually to the profit of someone's wallet. A shortlist of some of those ideas could be:

"It's really difficult to lose weight and chances of success are limited"

"No pain, no gain"

"Losing weight requires an enormous amount of willpower and motivation"

"To lose weight you have to go down the path of most-resistance"

"You have to cut down on your food and eat less to lose weight"

"It takes a really long time to lose weight"

"It's best to lose weight slowly (anyway) so as not to cause any adverse effects in the body"

And my personal favourite, which was told to a friend of mine by a surgeon who was about to remove 2/3 of my friend's stomach with a "bypass" operation:

"Even if you do lose weight, your body, your cells, are now programmed to be 'fat' so no matter what you do you will ultimately put the weight back on to bring you back to that weight, if not heavier"

Glancing through these phrases, and I'm sure you can think up many more, how do they make you feel? For years I had those sentences turning around in my mind, which made losing weight feel really hard, I felt that I was going to fail before even trying. It's disheartening to think that we are going to put ourselves through a huge inner struggle, 24/7, for something that we are told is "incurable" anyway?

But what if we were to replace those phrases by the **Truth?**

"It's really difficult to lose weight and chances of success are limited?"
"It's just as easy to lose weight as it is to put it on"
It took me over three years to go from 54kg to 93.5kg, it took me under eight months to lose that same weight. I'm not alone in having attained that kind of result.

"No pain, no gain?"
"When you are lighter, you will be in far less pain and will have gained a whole lot – and getting there is easy"
I can assure you that any pain you may have now, due to the weight that you're carrying around, will dissipate – joint pains, sciatica, headaches, digestive ailments. I find it almost shameful that people, who are already in pain, physically and psychologically, are being told that they have to endure even more pain in order to reach their health. Here is how I simplify it – pain and health are not synonymous, they are antonymous, so how can one reasonably justify going through pain, physical and mental, in order to gain health. Pain is tantamount to dis-ease; it's that simple.

"Losing weight requires an enormous amount of willpower and motivation?"
"Losing weight doesn't require any more motivation or willpower than putting on weight does"

Does a 'thin' person require motivation and willpower to say no to a cake? The only thing that distinguishes you from a 'thin' person is your own belief-system and thinking around your own self-image.

When I think back to when I was obese, I can say in all honesty that it required far more motivation and willpower to eat that cake, or that pork pie, or that packet of crisps, than I ever required when I just simply stopped doing it. If you look at the mechanism, you know that by eating those things you're damaging your body and that deep down the only thing you really want is health. Despite this you still force food, which you know is not good for you, into your mouth, following that by a period of harsh mental self-flagellation. That!, my friends, requires enormous motivation and willpower.

"To lose weight you have to go down the path of most-resistance?"
"By going down the path of least-resistance, you will attain your goals far more easily"
When you take the pressure off, whether it is on the nutritional level or in any other area of your life, it suddenly becomes so easy - you just breeze through things. Again, nobody wants to live with a 24/7 struggle, it's not a natural way of living. When you take the pressure off, you also quiet the thoughts around losing weight.

During the months when I dropped the 45 kilos or so, I wasn't thinking or obsessing about weight loss. I did recognize the positive changes that I could feel and see, but the part where I would continuously beat myself up was gone. I took a very simple approach to food, which made it really easy. I didn't have to resist any kinds of foods because if I did eat them it wasn't a big deal and I would just go back to my normal eating habits at the next meal. There was no taboo on food so I actually lost all interest in the "bad" foods as they weren't important. I had less thinking around food, which enabled me to reprioritise my life and focus more on my children, my husband, my work, my friends, etc.

"You have to cut down on your food and eat less to lose weight?"
"You have to eat more healthily to lose weight and know how to organize your eating"
Again, here we have the popular misconception that privation and suffering is necessary for losing weight and leading a healthier lifestyle. Now, I'm not saying that you should overeat, but I am saying that you have to eat enough, as we discussed in part 1. I remember a friend of mine, who was considerably taller than I am, once accused me of overeating because I was eating more than they were. In considering my friend's statement, I first looked at how I was physically and emotionally at the time. Despite eating more than that other person, I was in good shape, had lots of energy and felt good in myself. When I compared the plates, sure, there was more food on my plate but they were not the same foods as on my friend's plate. In fact I did eat more but I ate more in quality and nutritional value. Once more, losing weight and eating healthily has nothing to do with the amount that you eat and everything to do with the quality of what you eat.

"It takes a really long time to lose weight?"
"You can lose weight at the speed that you wish – it's up to you"
Through personal experience I know that weight loss can be very rapid but I believe that what is most important is how you feel. It's ultimately up to you. I have clients who prefer making gradual changes and I have others who prefer going the whole hog and changing everything immediately. In both cases, the results are there. Often what I do find is that those who start out with a gradual change in mind, very quickly ask

me to help them put into place a more rapid change when they see how easy it is to do. As I said before, you can lose weight just as rapidly as you can put it on.

Making changes in your eating habits is not hard at all; it's as easy as pie (pun intended!) If, for some reason, you had to change the locks on your front door, and the new lock turned to the left, rather than the right, within a day you would have adapted. The brain registers quickly how to do things. It won't take you six months to integrate the new way of turning the lock to the left. The only thing that can stop you changing it is if you start telling yourself that it's hard, hyper-complicated, too "techy", etc. The barrier to changing the way of unlocking the door comes from thought, not from the new lock. Recognizing the way thought works is the key to not allowing it to be a barrier.

"It's best to lose weight slowly (anyway) so as not to cause any adverse effects in the body?"
"It's best to lose weight as soon as possible"
Your body is neither programmed to eat unhealthily nor to drag excess weight around. The honest truth is, the longer you eat unhealthily and the longer you have an excess of weight, the bigger the toll will be on your long-term health.

Telling people that they should lose weight slowly adds to the idea that it's hard, that it's a long struggle. I've not met anyone yet who, being overweight, has not wished to lose that weight as rapidly as possible; who would not dearly love to wake up the next morning and find it miraculously gone. This is one of the main reasons that people attempt extreme solutions for weight loss, from taking expensive pills to medical interventions and surgery.

My friend, who had the stomach bypass, actually lost half of her body weight in six months. The surgeons never said that the weight loss was too rapid, in fact they were actually "very pleased" with her "progress"! And just in case you are considering that kind of operation as a possible solution; the surgeons basically removed my friend's stomach so that any food she ate passed immediately through her system, in one end – out the other, and the vitamins and minerals that she is now unable to assimilate have to be ingested through supplementary pills made up of artificial, chemically manufactured nutrients. She eats a smaller meal than my children did when they were babies and, as babies, the food has to be somewhat liquefied, as the stomach is no longer there to deal with the solid foods. She also has to take a whole pile of medication to counteract an overproduction of bile that could burn her oesophagus and what's left of her intestine, other pills to combat diarrhoea, others to regulate the heart, kidney and liver functions, others to regulate the cholesterol levels.

"Even if you do lose weight, your body, your cells, are now programmed to be 'fat' so no matter what you do you will ultimately put the weight back on to bring you back to that weight, if not heavier?"

"Your body is programmed for health"

Psychological and physical health is our default setting. To lead people to believe that even if they finally lose the weight, the results will be short-lived and that they will end up back at square one is absolutely outrageous. The only thing that can make us put the weight back on is to return to our unhealthy eating habits. The body is NOT programmed to be overweight and it is NOT a fatality! The surgeon who said that to my friend, in order to manipulate her into going through a potentially dangerous and expensive operation has lessened her quality of life, not only from a nutritional point of view but also because as she still lives with the internal psychological struggle of weight loss, despite having lost a huge amount.

I lost the weight six years ago; I have not put it back on. It fluctuates a little depending on how I eat at different periods but I'm just a normal weight now and living physically and psychologically in the way that Nature intended.

The Problem with Diet Labels

Our capacity to verbalize neural impulses in our brain is a wonderful and miraculous thing. It has allowed us to develop tools, invent new ways of doing things, cultivate, explore – it has allowed us to survive. The curse of this verbal capacity is that it has brought us to a place where we believe that we are superior beings to all other living creature on the planet and, as such, we have forgotten somewhat that we are part of Nature and not separate from it. The upside to our linguistic capacities is that we can name things and make them more easily recognizable, the words aid us in navigating through our surroundings – whether those words are in our heads as thought or vocalized outwardly. The downside is that we have forgotten that the words are just there to help us navigate; once we have given something a name, we then take ownership of it and begin to surround that "name" with other meanings – this can lead to good and bad.

These surrounding meanings are nothing more than supplementary thoughts that we consider reality – beliefs and rules. As human beings, we make rules all the time and as soon as we have taken ownership of something through naming it, we start making up a whole set of rules around it. You only have to look at a law book to see the mechanism. Take any article of law and you will find accompanying that article (rule) a whole set of additional clauses (rules) and some of them in complete contradiction with the original article.

The thing with us human being is, though we make rules

all the time, we don't actually much like living by rules, not any more than any other living creature on the planet. Could you imagine the birds passing a law saying that no bird has the right to fly between 12pm and 2pm? How many birds do you think would respect that? In the same way the bird is free to spread its wings and fly whenever he wishes to, human beings yearn to be able to spread our wings and fly whenever we wish to. Thus, the more rules we make, the less free we feel and the more we go against the natural order.

This is the reason that, when I decided to write this book, I refused the idea of putting a name and calling it the "such-and-such diet". For, every single "title" diet out there comes with a whole set of rules. You're allowed to eat this, but not that except at this time of the day, when that's okay but you'd better not make a regular habit of it for fear of suffering "such-and-such" a consequence if you do." Whoa! Small wonder we can't handle it without feeling frustrated and deprived. These diets contain scrolls of rules that you have to remember. The number of times I've done a mid-afternoon face palm when I've suddenly remembered that "SH**! I wasn't supposed to eat that at lunchtime!" There is no title, no ownership of my suggestions here because there are no rules.

I was discussing with a client recently who "admitted" to me that he had "started" but then "stopped." So I asked him "what did you start and what did you stop? If there are no rules, there is nothing to start or stop" He was afraid that I would be judgemental but if there are no rules, there is nothing to judge and as a side note, who the heck am I to judge anyone anyway?
As far as dieting is concerned, if there are no rules, there are no rules to break. If there is no "title" diet, then there is no diet to break and when there is no diet to break, there is no pressure, no feelings of guilt, no beating yourself up, no feeling bad about yourself, no feelings of lack of self-worth, no feelings of being a loser, no

feelings of not being good enough, no feelings of being abnormal.

Does the "healthy" person beat himself up for having had a cake? Does he say to himself "oh no, what a disaster! I shouldn't have done that!" No! Of course not! It's just part and parcel of everyday living. Why should it be any different for you? You're just the same as everyone else on this planet. There's nothing wrong with you. Why should you make up all these rules around eating and, moreover, make that so hard for yourself?

When I was obese, I already knew what to do in order to lose weight. I already knew how the biochemistry works, how different foods affect our body. I knew why I had put on weight and I knew why I wasn't losing it. So, with the knowledge, why on earth did I wait ten years before doing something about it? The answer is simple; I was making up rules, rules that clipped my wings. That famous day when I got up and decided not to try any more, the day that everything changed, was the day I stopped making up rules. From that day I gave myself the freedom to fly.

Health – The Default Setting

There are stories the world over and stories as old as time about people who have been diagnosed with incurable conditions, terminal illnesses that have gone through seemingly miraculous recoveries, recoveries that baffle doctors and scientists. How can that be?

Our bodies are made up of cells, molecules, particles, atoms, electrons, protons, etc. Not only do our brains think, but our cells also "think" and they communicate within the body – this is where intuition comes from. We have millions of years of cellular programming that will help us in our quest to return to health. Listening to that internal communication and tuning into that age-old Wisdom will us naturally what to do.

If you can imagine a computer (our body) running on a perfect operating system (health) that is as old as time itself. On that computer we are running other programmes (our eating habits). However, some of the newer programmes are not adapted to the original operating system and so, the operating system will send up an error message (weight gain and food-related ailments). Here we have a choice: we can continue to run the new programme despite the adverse effects on the operating system or we can choose to employ a programme that is more appropriate to what the computer needs to run on, to keep in line with the original fabric (Nature).

When you tune into your body, tune into that operating system, you will see and feel the signs when something is amiss in your eating habits. Those signs will go from something as harmless as intestinal gas to serious ailments such as diabetes and heart disease. But it's never too late to change the programme you're running given your body's health default setting. Now, the idea is not to say "ah, there's such and such going on in my body, I'm falling ill" and then to make up a set of rules, but to listen to what is happening in order to find a more accurate approach, based on intuition.

If I can give a specific example: when your body is producing too much insulin, you are going to have symptoms of irritability, tiredness, craving sweet or high salt foods, dizziness, and generally the feeling of a "need" to eat. One of the worst things you can possibly do in that case is to refuse your body food, yet that is what we have been taught that we should do and, to add to that, we are even told that not only should we not eat, we should go off and exercise for an hour or two. We are putting an enormous strain on our body when we could simply respond to its need, especially considering that the longer you "hold off" the greater tendency you will have to eat something "unhealthy." How can we possibly hope that our bodies can cope with such unnatural behaviour? Of course our operating system is going to send out a ton of error messages.

The good news is that as soon as you are running the programmes that are appropriate for our perfect operating system, the error messages rapidly disappear; it's just a question of running the programme that's in harmony with the system.

Scientists have recently brought forth evidence that the Universe functions in the same manner as a giant brain with the neural activity among brain cells being mirrored by the shape of expanding galaxies. This doesn't surprise me in the slightest as we are made up of all the same elements. We are, metaphorically, joined at the hip or rather the heart. The energy of life is infinite in ways that we are unable to fathom for, even if we are mortal in our bodies, Nature is everlasting because space-time is infinite and we are of that infinite energy. The Universe is programmed for life and is living. That alone proves for me the default health setting; how could it be otherwise?

we are programmed to be healthy + vibrant.

The Power of Thought

"When you start to see the power of Thought and its relationship to your way of observing life, you will better understand yourself and the world in which you live"
Sydney Banks, The Missing Link

So the big question is this – How do you move into this new mindset? Traditionally we are told that we have to deliberately make ourselves do it, which brings us back to the factors of motivation and willpower. What if there were a far easier and a far gentler manner of going about it?

Of course, you have the choice as to which method you want to work with; if your way is the motivation/willpower way then that is your way, but if you change your mind, here is another approach that I will illustrate with this example.

A friend of mine decided to take the hard-slog path and I completely respect his choice. However, I have seen him write several times around the themes of "resistance" "struggling" "tiredness" "headaches" "bad moods" and general feelings of low self-esteem. One evening he wrote the following statement: "it is only right to say that after this weekend.... I am a complete failure!!" I queried this last statement and he replied that his only redeeming feature was that he had been able to resist chocolate. It's very sad that a person making so much effort should feel that bad about themselves.

But here's the thing, "failure" is just a thought isn't it? Whatever happens to be going on that meaning can only exist if we decide it. We have infinite possibility for any kind of new thought to come at any moment (we have something between 70 000 to 120 000 thoughts every day.) No matter what your thoughts happen to be about, good or bad, those thoughts will eventually pass and leave space for some new thought. Thought is temporary in nature but we can get stuck in our thoughts when we indulge in them. If we have negative thoughts such as "I'm a complete failure," and we understand that the thought will pass, we don't take it quite so seriously, in recognizing it for what it is... a Thought. But if we are not aware of that then we can easily get trapped in our negative thinking and end up feeling profoundly unhappy.

The psychiatrist and Three Principles teacher, Dr. Bill Pettit, explains that it only takes 3 to 5 minutes of negative thinking to negatively affect the brain chemistry, creating a low state of mind. Once we are in that low state of mind, we are more prone to having negative thoughts. The more we pursue that negative thinking and indulge in it, the more the brain chemistry is affected and this can lead to serious depression. At the same time, by putting additional strain on our brain and body chemistry through restrictive or unhealthy eating, we end up with a super potent cocktail of sadness that can seem impossible to escape from.

Just to be very clear, this is not a question of positive thinking or doing affirmations. Deliberate positive thinking and affirmations actually contribute to ill ease and can lead to even deeper levels of depression. When there is a voice in the head saying "I'm rubbish at everything I do and I'm the world's biggest loser ever!" (That's my own personal favourite) and you fight it off with "I'm a wonderful person and getting better at what I do every day and I'm a winner" you are actually sending mixed messages through your brain, affecting the chemistry in a way that the brain is not meant to cope with. And believe me, that irresolvable internal conflict can be endless if you pursue it.

Feeling down, feeling rubbish, stupid, ugly, unlovable, (and many other negative emotions) are simply part of the human experience, just as we can feel elated, fantastic, clever, beautiful and lovable. We are taught however that we are not supposed to have negative emotions and that there is something wrong with us when we do have them. We are told that it's due to our upbringing, our education, our parents and so it goes on, and that we have to resolve this negativity by consulting doctors, psychologists, psychiatrists whilst taking medication. On the other hand, we are also taught that too much positive thinking is also bad. We shouldn't overdo the positives lest we become bigheaded/full of ourselves/selfish. How on earth are we supposed to find our true nature when we have such conflicting messages?

If we can only see that ALL emotions are perfectly normal and natural and that they are coming from our own thinking, then we realize that we don't have to make such a big deal out of them. It's funny to note that despite all the affirmations and positive thinking, there are more depressed people in our society today than ever before. By simply seeing and understanding that we are in a low state of mind, that our level of consciousness has dropped and that we are somewhat caught up in our thinking, then that thinking will simply pass and give way to something new. With that understanding we become aware that no matter what the 'thought-feeling' state, our well being is still present; the awareness of the illusion of our thinking can bring us instant peace of mind.

This was precisely my experience when it came to food and my eating habits; I just stopped fixating on the negatives. If I had eaten a cake I just said to myself "so what!" I didn't feel the need to make a big deal of it. If I started to beat myself up, I would just notice that that's what I was doing and would recognize that what I had eaten was also affecting my body chemistry and increasing the level of negative thinking, which in a short time would pass.

Not getting stuck in my thinking meant two things: firstly, I would simply continue my normal eating habits at the next meal. Secondly, that very rapidly foods I had labelled up until then as "bad" foods lost that label and meaning; the importance that I had been giving to that meaning disappeared because I could see that I had been the one always deciding that meaning and importance. With no more taboo, there was no need for resistance or beating up myself up! I didn't have to fight any more, the battle against the kilos was, and still is, relinquished.

This is my hope for you, that you can find the way to

making it easy to lose weight because it's not hard. When we can see through the thought mechanisms that are going on, whether personally or on a larger scale, then we can simply let go. When you see that the things that you say about yourself are just thoughts and nothing more, your life will change. Your thoughts will, at some point in the future (and it may be only a second from now), give way to new thoughts. Once we understand this then we don't have to take our thoughts so seriously. Imagine three months from now: you've lost some weight and/or you're simply feeling better through some simple effortless changes in your eating habits – are you still going to be having those thoughts?

This potential for new thought, and being aware of that potential, is how you are going to help yourself out of this situation that you feel so stuck in. My own personal experience and the experiences of the people I have helped thus far, is proof of that. You don't need years of analysis to understand your relationship with food; you simply have to become aware of your thinking and that, my dear friends, is so easy.

Sure, there are times when I still get lost in my thinking but when I remember the nature of thought, I catch myself and say "Ah, got stuck in my thinking again! Oh darn!" Understanding the mechanism is all the insight you will need to be able to let go of it. This understanding, believe me will have a wonderful effect on your life, not just on your physical health, since our thought mechanism colours every aspect of our lives. How wonderful is that?

"Whatever thought you have tomorrow that really troubles you, will not trouble you as much at some time in the future. If you knew that at the time, imagine what a difference it would make. The principles is the answer to the "how do I know?" at the time. As you understand at a deeper and deeper level, you recognize earlier and earlier "this too shall pass", this is just thought and I'll get over it. Then you get new thought and new thought presents the situation differently and in a nicer way. If you have a thought like "I haven't accomplished enough in my life" you may have a new thought that says "what is enough, how do you define enough?" You might have the thought "actually I have accomplished something" but all of these thoughts are transitory too" - George Pransky, Tikun Conference "New Discoveries In Psychology That Make Well Being More Accessible"

Part 2b

The Practicalities
of
The Mind-Body Connection

A Combination for Success

"Breakfast: Hot-cross bun (Scarsdale diet - slight variation on specified piece of wholemeal toast); Mars bar (Scarsdale diet - slight variation on specified half grapefruit)

Snack: two bananas, two pears (switched to F-plan as starving and cannot face Scarsdale carrot snacks). Carton orange juice (Anti-Cellulite Raw-Food diet)

Lunch: jacket potato (Scarsdale vegetarian diet) and hummus (Hay diet - fine with jacket spuds as all starch, and breakfast and snack were all alkaline-forming with exception of hot-cross bun and Mars: minor aberration)

Dinner: four glasses of wine, fish and chips (Scarsdale Diet and also Hay diet - protein forming); portion tiramisu; peppermint Aero (pissed)"

Bridget Jones's Diary, p.74 - by Helen Fielding

So we have seen and spoken much about how the psychological state and the physiological state are strongly linked together; both affect the biochemistry of the body and thus, both affect moods. How many of you have noticed that when in a low-state of mind you tend to not care about how you eat, you perhaps go for the "unhealthier" types of foods? Often these are the foods that have a high sugar/salt/fat content that negatively affects the biochemistry, increasing the low state of mind. Thus, you find yourself, momentarily, in a higher state of mind through the food intake but ultimately in a lower state of mind once those elements have gone through your body. Low state of mind ----->"Unhealthy food"----->Higher State of Mind----->Lower-State of Mind. This is how I ate myself in all innocence all the way to a whopping 180 pounds/93.5kg/14st.

It's important to know that those "extreme" foods with

high sugar, fat, salt content, release endorphins in the brain, thus the "quick fix". Once the quick fix is over, the endorphins decrease and can even drop lower. In the same way as the pancreas doesn't "understand" what's happening because these "unhealthy" foods are not naturally found in nature and ends up malfunctioning, so does the pituitary gland that produces the endorphins. We end up with insulin and endorphin resistance and then both systems pack up.

It is a little bit a case of "which came first, the chicken or the egg?" Did I start eating in the way that I did because, initially, I was in a low state of mind or did the food I was eating create the low-state of mind? All I can say is that it was a downwards spiral. When you realize within yourself that, whether it be what I call "socially accepted comfort eating" or the worst possible eating disorder - the origin is always the same:

We are looking for an external solution to an inner problem and we do it in all innocence.

The reason for your low state of mind is inside and not outside yourself. Your own thinking, whether triggered by biochemistry or not, is what's creating the low state of mind and therefore anything outside of yourself is not going to "fix" the problem. You don't have to eat that food any more to make yourself feel better because you already have the power within you to feel better. Our default setting is health and well being, both physical and mental.

Time to Eat

"Cooking is like love. It should be entered into with abandon or not at all"
Harriet Van Horne

"One cannot think well, love well, sleep well, if one has not dined well"
Virginia Woolf

A popular expression tells us that we should "breakfast as a king, lunch as a prince and dine as a peasant". I used to believe that referred to the amount that I was eating: that we needed to eat a large quantity of food in the morning and only a small amount of food in the evening. The problem was that I was never hungry enough to have a large amount of food in the morning, which left me feeling hungry mid-morning. In the evening I would eat around 6pm, but after 10pm my tummy would be rumbling, making it difficult to get to sleep.

When I started out on my weight loss journey, it suddenly dawned on me that what that expression meant was that richer foods are better in the morning and lighter foods later on in the evening. "Richer foods" have a higher protein and fat content and "lighter foods" contain less protein and have a lower fat content. I was very happy with this realization as this meant that a traditional English breakfast was back on the menu if I so desired it, although, due to my understanding of the role of insulin, I dropped the fried bread and toast apart from the odd occasion.

Very naturally around lunchtime I was finding myself more attracted to the darker meats or the more oily fish, which take longer to digest, so I tend to have those richer "meats" at midday.

In the evening I have the whiter meats and fish that have less protein and fat or I have wholegrain rice/spelt flour pasta with vegetables. Other times, if I'm not feeling particularly hungry I have fruit in the evening followed by some dark chocolate with 70% cocoa. I will have the rice and pasta, after all I enjoy them, but I do keep the GI content of these foods low and this balances the protein. On the odd occasion I will have the starch that has a higher GI but since my body is no longer over-producing insulin, they don't have the same adverse effect that they would have done in the past.

A lot of diets speak about the alkaline-acid content of food and though I've not studied that closely, it seems to me that there may be some truth in that. When I mix starch foods with animal protein, and more so when the starch foods have a higher GI, I end up with a more or less serious gastric reaction, often feeling sluggish after the meal. That's the basic reason that I don't mix animal protein and anything starchy, though I still make Spaghetti Bolognese, Cassoulet (a French dish consisting of haricot beans in a tomato and goose fat sauce served with duck/sausage), or Lentils with sausages and similar dishes. Whatever I happen to be eating, I simply bear in mind the 'quality content' but taking the quality content into account doesn't mean that I make up a rule around that and force myself to exclude things from my diet that I might otherwise enjoy.

Similarly, I encourage you to be mindful of the amount of sugar/glucose intake in your diet, again not to eliminate it completely, that would be no fun but merely to be conscious of what you're eating so that you have a greater choice.

Exercise - What It's Really Good For

"The joy of life consists in the exercise of one's energies, continual growth, constant change, the enjoyment of every new experience.
To stop means simply to die.
The eternal mistake of mankind is to set up an attainable ideal"
Aleister Crowley

We are constantly told that we have to eat less and exercise more. Yet you know how difficult it is to get up and exercise when you feel so heavy that you have difficulty putting your shoes on – I used to get out of breath just getting dressed in the morning – or if you are really hungry with symptoms of hypoglycaemia.

The truth of the matter is that exercise alone will not help you lose weight. Yes, it has a favourable effect on the metabolism and can calm the insulin production. It also releases endorphins in the brain that will give you that "feel good" sensation. However, if you continue to eat "unhealthy" foods you won't be seeing the results that you are hoping for.

Another important element to take into account is that if you are heavy, you're going to be putting extra stress on your joints and bones, particularly if you are not in the habit of exercising. I, personally, waited until I'd lost 20 – 25kg before I attempted exercise, first of all to safeguard my joints and secondly because I didn't feel that I had the energy to exercise up until that point.

Now, I'm not saying that we should just sit at home and not do anything but I am saying that if we're not in the habit of exercising then this should be approached really quite gently. When I had got to the point where I felt that I was able to exercise and, moreover, wanted to, I started with cycling and swimming. Both of those activities offer support to your framework and are also inexpensive.

The most important aspect of exercise is not the exercise itself – it's the fact that when you are exercising you are clearing your mind and allowing the possibility for fresh and new creative thought to come through.

When I'm out cycling for example, I'm looking at nature and breathing it in. I'm watching the sun come up or set. I'm breathing fresh air. I'm listening to the birds singing. I'm feeling the rain on my skin and making enormous splashes through puddles. What I'm doing is not exercising, what I'm doing is allowing my physical body to get back in tune with Nature, allowing my Spirit to have a little fun, allowing my thoughts to slow down. I don't have to push myself to do it; I don't have to force myself out. I want and appreciate those moments of solitude where I can just be.

We have a tendency to believe that if we don't push and/or force ourselves to do something NOW that we will never do it. That is supposing that the thought to actually go and do exercise will never pop up in your mind, and if we don't force ourselves we are deemed lazy and weak. What if your lack of desire to exercise is coming from your own inner wisdom that is telling you that it's not the right time? We are so busy attempting to make things happen, to pursue goals, that we forget that we can just allow things to unfold naturally and gently, that there is no need for us to control everything.

When you are in a place of calm, with a clear head, you have far more chance of achieving what you desire than if you are living in constant stress and pain with a clouded perception of your environment; incapable of tapping into your inner wisdom.

By all means exercise but exercise in a manner that is enjoyable to you. If you enjoy dancing, go and dance, if you like team sports, go and do that. If you enjoy pulling weights at the gym then go and do that. But only do it if you enjoy it and each and every one of us has some kind of physical activity that we enjoy. Nobody says that it has to be hard, only your thoughts say that.

Walking, if that's all you feel capable of, is one of the most easy and enjoyable types of exercise. It takes you outside, gets some air in your lungs, improves your heart rate and, even though considered so moderate an exercise to almost be rejected, it will help regulate your metabolism and the insulin production - combine that with a new set of eating habits and you won't even need to think about what you're doing, it will just be very natural.

Throw Away the Scales

I'm talking about the bathroom kind not about the kitchen kind. Though I never weigh my food in basic meals, if I'm making a cake or a particular recipe, the kitchen scales maintain their utility.

Why throw away the bathroom scales? In order to also throw away the associated pressure, stress and need for motivation and willpower that we associate with losing weight. We have in our society a myth of an "ideal weight", based on a number. We have in our minds that we "should" weigh such and such, so we become obsessive and, if you're anything like me, ended up weighing yourself three to four times a day, simply in the hope of seeing an improvement for all that effort – ah, the disappointment! An ideal weight is when you feel healthy and able to do all the things that you want to do and when you feel comfortable in your clothes, not a number.

Some use the Body Mass Index (BMI) to measure themselves, but the BMI rating is a generalized index and, though it is a pretty good indication, I don't believe that it should be written in stone. The BMI also fails to take into account the fact that muscle mass weighs more than the adipose mass, which can make you think that you are doing something wrong and are failing (when you are not). A woman, a few days before her period, can put on up to 3kg through water retention – the BMI doesn't take that into account either. What I'm saying is that the number of kilos and the BMI category that you enter into are simply an indication and not a golden rule. Being thin is not an indication of health, *feeling healthy in mind and body* is an indication of health.

Easy Eating

In our modern day society we have come to a conclusion that we don't have time to make and prepare food. We get home from work exhausted, maybe we feel we've had a bad day and the last thing we feel like doing is preparing a meal from scratch – it's much easier just to open the freezer and put something tasty in the oven while we check our e-mails. Now that's true and I'm all for ready-made meals but of the homemade kind.

One of the simplest methods of cooking is with a steam cooker and you can cook practically anything in it. If you happen to have one with a timer you can put your food into the steam baskets, switch it on and go and relax. The preparation time isn't any longer than putting a ready-made meal in the oven or making a sandwich.

I like to keep my food down to basics, except on special occasions where I will make more elaborate meals. By using the basics, it is quick and easy and also inexpensive, and in any case certainly not any more expensive than the ready-made items.

Another option is to make large portions of whatever it is you're cooking, which will give you meals in advance that you can freeze yourself, for example. Thus, when you get home during the week, "tired", having had a "bad day" and "not feeling like cooking," you have a natural-ingredients ready made meal that just needs heating up. We have refrigerators, freezers, microwave ovens, steam cookers, pressure cookers – everything is there making it easy for us to cook simply and quickly but, and again I'm going to blame the media for this, we think that it's too much trouble because we are constantly bombarded with images telling us so. Surely we are more intelligent than that? In reality, reheating something you've made in advance is, well, a piece of cake! The main advantage is that you know exactly what you are putting into the dish – there are no surprises with basic ingredients.

Of course it does require a little organization and a little planning in advance. Very often I make the meals up on the Sunday before the start of the week, it doesn't take more time to make several meals in one go, and I either freeze or refrigerate the dishes depending on how quickly they perish.

There are two other reasons why I make food this way: they are "economical" and "ecological". I re-use, recycle what is already there which costs less and I don't have huge amounts of packaging to throw away.

To give you an idea of the price for one week's shopping, imagining that all my cupboards and fridge/freezer are bare, and including breakfast and the "extras" that I buy for my children. This could be and example shopping list:

Clementines	Morteau sausage	Butter
Apples	Minced beef	Goat's Cheese
Tomatoes	Duck	Milk
Savoy Cabbage	Chicken	Mineral water
Leeks	Eggs (organic)	
Celery		
Courgettes	Pure orange juice	
Aubergines	Pure apple juice	
Mushrooms	Pure lemon juice	
Garlic	Tea - green and black	
Onions		

Spelt flour pasta	Frozen green beans
Haricot beans	Frozen broccoli
Wholegrain rice	Frozen salmon fillets
Dried split peas	Frozen white fish
Organic lentils	Tins of tomatoes
Spelt flour	
Porridge oats	Chocolate biscuits
Yeast	Dark chocolate
Olive oil	Dried raisins

So, if I had absolutely no food in the house and needed to stock up, this is what I would buy. Obviously here, I've only given the example with food, as like everyone else, I need to buy toothpaste and toilet paper and a few cleaning products! Also, what's important to bear in mind is that not all of this food would be used in a week and this is based on a shopping basket for a family of four.

The total price for 41 items is €140/$184/£113, making an average price per item of €3.40/$4.50/£2.75
(All prices are approximate, based on French shops, Spring 2013)

When I compare this average price range to the prices of a well-known French supermarket's own brand of readymade meals I find this (prices in euros):

A 600g family size pizza will cost €2.99

800g worth of mini-Quiche Lorraines will cost €3.99

A 1Kg family size Lasagne or Shepherd's Pie will cost €2.58

A 1kg bag of Paëlla will cost €3.76

A 1kg bag of Pasta with Chicken and Vegetables will cost €3.99

Most French families will start a meal with a soup, bought in a carton, and these soups range (for a one litre carton) in price from €0.90 to €1.95, for the shop's own brand, or from €1.55 to €3.50 for one of the more well known brands.

Most French families will also finish their meal with some kind of dessert, usually some type of yoghurt or milk based dessert. These desserts range from roughly €0.14-€0.20, for the shop's own brand, to €0.21-€0.27 per pot for the more expensive brands.

Not forgetting €0.85 on average for the traditional white baguette.

So an average evening meal for a French family of four, two adults and two children would cost between €5.30/$7.00/£4.33 and €9.42/$12.45/£7.70

If I calculate the average price of a meal with my own example shopping list I get a cheaper deal of around €5.00/$6.60/£4.09

Given that my average weekly shopping costs around €80/$105/£65, the average price for a meal is more in the region of €2.85/$3.75/£2.33

How does that compare to your own weekly shopping budget?

Hungry or Hypoglycaemia

This is probably one of the easiest aspects to work out but where so many of us can get lost. To know which is which you have to be very clear and in tune with your body. Hungry is easy to know – your stomach is grumbling, you may be feeling a little bit shaky, dizzy if you've gone past the lunchtime bell. A grumbling stomach is normal and the very sure physical sign from your body telling you that you are in need of food. There is only one thing to do in that case... and that is eat.

Hypoglycaemia (low blood sugar) however is a little bit sneakier. The obvious signs are: dizziness; shakiness; and blurred vision but there can also be far less obvious signs: headaches; tiredness; yawning; feeling low; and irritability. The problem, of course, is that we may well have a tendency to blame those latter feelings on outside elements. Too much time in front of the computer screen gives us a headache; having worked too hard can create tiredness and yawning; problems with work colleagues or at home creates feelings of being low and irritable. These outer elements can appear very real but the fact of the matter is, particularly if you have eaten high GI foods, that those feelings may well be the result of hypoglycaemia, which is negatively effecting your mood and subsequently your thinking. It is a vicious circle: low blood sugar results in a low feeling or mood, which you blame on your environment, making you feel even worse.

So what to do? Well, in all honesty, if you are in a state of hypoglycaemia, the solution is the same as when you are hungry: you need to eat something.

My suggestion is that you eat something that has a low GI. Eating a chocolate bar or a bag of crisps will get you out of the low blood sugar but will ultimately put you back there in the hour or two that follows.

Unfortunately, depending on the level of the low blood sugar we are going to be more or less attracted to those high GI foods – it's a quick fix but one that creates a long term problem and will, if we keep at it, create long term illness. Of course, the best idea is to avoid getting into that state in the first place!

The Truth about the Glycemic Index

The Glycemic Index (GI) is the indicator of the level of sugar (glucose) in the blood after food intake, measured in g/per litre. The measurement is formed from the GI of sugar taken after fasting, which is 100.

We've all heard of the terms "slow sugars" and "rapid sugars" and we have been led to believe for many years now that the type of carbohydrate consumed does not effect the blood sugar levels. The traditional paradigm teaches us that some carbohydrates will be absorbed more quickly than others; this was based on the molecular structure of the carbohydrate i.e. simple molecular structures including simple sugar, honey, fruit, which would be absorbed rapidly and complex molecular structures including cereals, pulses, roots, which would be absorbed over a longer period going up to several hours.

The theory, according to this model, is that the rapid sugars will then be more readily available to give immediate energy, glucose, for the body, hence high glucose sports drinks; and the other carbohydrates will be absorbed more slowly, allowing a gradual energy release during the hours that follow food intake. Unfortunately, the body doesn't quite work that way and the above model is in fact not true. Generally speaking, the blood sugar levels will spike roughly twenty to thirty minutes after eating, and depending on what has been eaten, more or less glucose will be absorbed and is non-time related.

Let us compare two different types of carbohydrates, one with a high GI level to one that has a low GI level – white rice vs. lentils for example, both of which are considered to be complex slow acting sugars in the traditional nutrition method. The glucose in both of these types of foods is absorbed at the same speed but where the difference comes in is that the white rice will show a glucose spike of around 80 where the lentils will show a glucose spike of around 30.

What is interesting to note is that, following the white rice glucose spike, the blood sugars will fall very rapidly in comparison to the glucose spike following the lentils. Both will arrive around the 1g mark around the same time, as shown in the figure below. The resulting low blood sugar is clearly lower for the white rice than it is for the lentils. It's the difference between a calm sea and a choppy sea in our bodies... and minds.

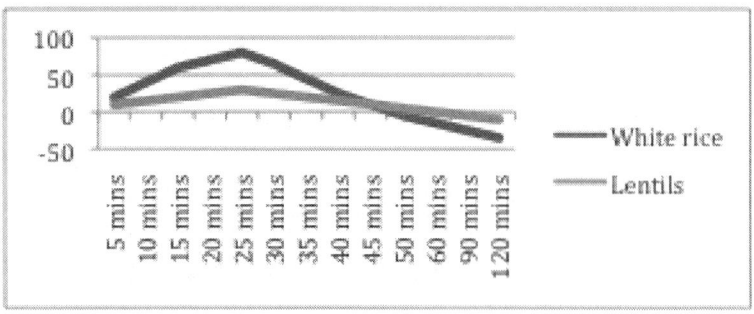

This graph is here purely as an example, the figures may not be scientifically exact.

The real question is why does it even matter and how does this help us? If you have a pancreas that is in perfect working order, in a sense it doesn't, at least as far as weight gain is concerned. However, if you have a tendency to put on weight easily, this information is of the greatest importance.

The higher the GI of a food, the more insulin you will

produce to cover the levels of glucose released; the insulin serves to regulate the blood glucose levels. The problems arise when the pancreas starts reacting badly to the constant bombardment of high glucose foods. Initially, the pancreas will start over-producing on insulin, simply because the human body is not designed to cope with that amount of glucose on a regular basis. The second problem arises when, despite, the insulin production, the glucose levels stay elevated, this is the state of insulin-resistance, which is very rapidly followed by a state of pre-diabetes leading to type II diabetes.

However, the obvious symptom of weight gain is not the only factor to be taken into account. Recent studies from Harvard have shown that, even in people who remain at what would be considered a healthy weight, there are increased factors of LDL cholesterol, elevated levels of triglycerides, high blood pressure, liver damage and heart conditions.
As I've mentioned before, weight is not systematically a sign of health, it can be a helpful indicator but is not a guarantee.

Generally speaking, food found in nature in it's natural untransformed state, and here I am talking about everything specifically vegetable, has a low glycemic index – most of the time, not going above a GI of around 35 and human beings, and all other animals who walk the earth, have been eating these low GI foods since their arrival on the planet.
We are the only species on earth, as far as I can tell, that have learned to manipulate the food that we eat, cook it, transform it, make it into something that it wasn't originally and now we are at the extreme where we add chemicals to our foods. Sure chemicals exist on earth but that doesn't mean that we necessarily should be eating them.
My children "mummy, mummied!" me one day into

buying them a packet of chocolate chip cookies, which I do buy for them but they are aware of the effects that those foods can have on their bodies from a long-term perspective and, in fact, they ask me for those foods less and less. In the chocolate chip cookies was ammonium carbonate. Now, I'm perfectly willing to accept that ammonium is already present in the human body but I'm not convinced that it's such a good idea to consume it directly into the digestive tract, but I digress.

What's important to take into account is that our cooking methods and all the other, even natural, transformation of foods that we undertake can contribute to a modification of the GI levels in the food.

Which brings me to the next point and one that should not be neglected.

We find in nature two types of food structure, specifically in the vegetable kingdom: food is either made up of fat and fibre or glucose and fibre. That doesn't necessarily mean that we should never eat fat and carbohydrate mixed together but I am attentive to the fact that if I do mix the two, then I will ensure that there is also a great amount of fibre included in the meal. For example if I am having steak and chips (fries), which combine animal protein and fat in the steak, plus a high GI carbohydrate with the potatoes, I will accompany that with fibrous foods such as mushrooms and a large salad.

However, though this may decrease the glucose absorption, more will get through than if I were to follow Nature's way and not mix the carbohydrate and the fat together in the first place, so I wouldn't recommend steak and chips on a daily basis, even with the salad and the mushrooms.

Another important point is how GI levels affect our bodies in different ways throughout the day. Now, this isn't really a problem if you are eating low GI foods but if you do decide to have, for example potatoes, I would recommend eating them around the midday mark. Why? First thing in the morning, a high glucose spike is probably not what is going to be the most useful for you. Your body is just waking up and has suddenly to deal with a whole bunch of glucose. This is not a great idea and will ultimately cause feelings of hunger, with dizziness and shakiness, around the mid-morning mark, and provoke the need to eat something (sweet) to stave off the resulting hypoglycaemia. At lunchtime, a meal high in GI carbohydrates may well leave you feeling sluggish in the afternoon. In the evening, high GI foods are more difficult to digest it and can leave you with a tendency to awaken the next morning feeling groggy and tired.

Again, generally speaking, I tend to keep the GI level in my food down; I just find it easier to deal with. I find there is so much choice in nature, such a wide variety of tastes, colours and flavours. White rice? Get out of here! Unless it's with sushi!

Here is a glycemic index table and shows the remarkable amount of choice we have in the foods simply found in Nature. I have listed some of the most commonly eaten foods and they are grouped from "Low"

☐ "Low to Medium" ☐ "Medium to High" ☐ "High"

Again, and I can't insist enough on this, this is not a rulebook, this is simply information so that you can make the best choices that you feel are right for you.

GI Table *(for information purposes only!)*

Low GI < = 15 to 35	Raw onions, garlic, broccoli, cauliflower, raw green beans, cabbage, celery, Brussels sprouts, courgettes, aubergines, tomatoes, leeks, kale, artichokes, avocado, spinach, sweet peppers, asparagus, cucumber, olives, mushrooms, fresh green peas, salad, lettuce, lentils, split peas, haricot beans, chick peas, wild rice, quinoa, bamboo shoots, herbs and spices, oranges, apples, red fruits, grapefruits, fresh figs, peaches, plums, dried apricots, custard apple, coconut, nuts, chocolate 70% cocoa minimum.
Low to Medium GI 35 - 50	Quince, unsweetened carrot juice, dried fig, plums/dried prunes, oats, coconut milk, cider (Brut), Kamut, Egyptian wheat, kidney/pinto beans, buckwheat, kasha, no-sugar peanut butter, chicory, pumpernickel, falafel (fava beans), spaghetti al dente, quinoa flour, unsweetened grapefruit juice, freshly squeezed homemade orange juice, unripe bananas, whole couscous, whole semolina, fresh grapes, green and red, fresh pineapple, Kamut bread, tinned peas, whole rye, whole bulgur wheat, cranberry, whole spelt, jam with no sugar, brown basmati rice, unsweetened pineapple juice, white basmati rice, fresh mango, Jerusalem artichoke, unsweetened apple juice, unsweetened muesli, fresh Kiwifruit, sweet potatoes, All Bran, rye crackers, fresh litchis, brown rice, unsweetened cranberry juice, macaronis, unsweetened muesli

Medium to High GI 50 - 70	Industrial mustard, fresh papaya, tinned fruit, bulgur wheat, grape juice, loquat, shortbread, red rice, sushi, manioc, ripe bananas, oatmeal/cooked oats, long-grain rice, melons, plain ice cream, chestnut, Camargue rice, honey, pearl barley, marmalade, whole-grain bread, unpeeled steamed potato, tamarind, corn, beet/beetroot, raisins, breadfruit, sorbet, maple syrup, yam, Chinese noodles, jam made with sugar, sucrose, tacos, chocolate bars, gnocchi, noodles, molasses, refined cereal, rusk, bagels, biscuits, brown sugar, white bread, rice bread, brioche, potato chips, millet, sodas, rutabaga, polenta/cornmeal, matzo bread, dates
High 70 <	Watermelon, squash/marrow, white lasagne, sweetened rice milk, doughnuts, waffles, pumpkin, sports drinks, mashed potatoes, white flour crackers, puffed rice, hamburger buns, popcorn, corn starch, white flour, white bread, instant rice, rice cake, rice pudding, celeriac, tapioca, parsnip, cornflakes, arrowroot, gluten-free white bread, potato flour, baked potatoes, rice flour, fried potatoes, maltodextrin, corn starch, modified starch, glucose, glucose syrup, wheat syrup, rice syrup, beer, high fructose corn syrup

As can be seen so easily from this table, the more a food is transformed and manufactured into something that it wasn't originally; the higher the GI becomes. For example, high fructose corn syrup is terrifyingly at the top of the GI scale with an alarming GI of 115! All the more terrifying that we find it as an additive in so many industrially packaged foods

It is also important to note that certain basic foods in the higher GI sections of the table – watermelon, squash, celeriac, parsnip, rutabaga and dates, although they have a high GI the total glucid content of these foods remains very low, less than 5%. Thus, the insulin response is going to be in correlation, as our blood sugar levels would not normally be over-affected by these foods.

On the opposite scale, a food that I did not include in this table is milk, mostly because of the reasons evoked earlier on in the book. Even though it has a low GI, the proteins in the milk provoke a strong insulin response.

Again, as we have said before, if in doubt try these foods by all means and see how you feel – if it's wrong for you, your body will quickly let you know and as long as we are listening to what our bodies have to say, we never have to search any further.

"To know what you prefer instead of humbly saying Amen to what the world tells you you ought to prefer, is to have kept your soul Alive"
~ Robert Louis Stevenson

Annexe

Superfoods

Mother Nature's Miraculous Gift of Life

"We are living in a world today where lemonade is made
from artificial flavours and furniture polish is made from
real lemon"
Alfred E. Newman

"A nickel will get you on the subway, but garlic will get
you a seat"
Old New York Proverb

I have to admit that I consider all foods to be Superfoods. Nature is so well constructed and has literally set the table with everything we could possibly need for our physical and mental health. In recent years have come to light certain foods that contain particularly nutritious properties; they contain a fantastic concentration of nutrients that have a profound impact on our bodies. Some of these foods are already well known; others are just being discovered.

My personal opinion on this is: as long as it's a basic natural food, that it isn't toxic, then it will do us no harm. Of course, from a health point of view, it's not sufficient just to eat these foods – if the rest of the menu is unhealthy then the benefits of these Superfoods are going to be far less noticeable.

There are so many foods out there that enter into the category of Superfoods. Many of them help to trigger healing physiological responses in the body – blood sugar regulation; protection against cancer; high blood pressure; heart disease and Type II Diabetes. They help the body to rid itself of free radicals, combat the ageing process, contribute to the healthy renewal of cells and contribute to healthy body functions. There are so many in fact, that it would require an entire separate book to talk about them all, and there are books dedicated wholly to this subject.

For the purposes of this book I would like to present four, three of which have rather exceptional qualities. The first Superfood that I would like to touch on is the egg, not so much that it has the exceptional qualities of the other three Superfoods, but because the egg has received over the last few decades some very bad press, largely undeservingly and I would just like to crack open the mystery surrounding this rather wonderful and nutritious food.

The Egg – Unscrambling the Myth

For years the humble egg has been under attack from various different scientific bodies and is once more under attack - goodness knows why! Media headlines across the Globe have recently set the fox among the chickens by creating renewed hype by stating, *"Eggs are as bad for your arteries as smoking"* - the media do like to scramble everything they get their quills on if they believe they have something to crow about; I admit the article ruffled my feathers a bit! Those that do not have the time to go further and research the full contents of the study will conclude that eggs are rotten! On the contrary - eggs are really good for our health but first let's take a look at the study.

The original title of this Canadian study carried out by the Doctors David Spence, David Jenkins and Jean Davignon from the University of Western Ontario, Canada, of which their results were published in several science magazines, from August 2012 before being distorted by the general media when they got their claws into it was, "Egg Yolk Consumption and Carotid Plaque" - so egg yolks specifically! The study was done in conjunction with the analysis of artery damage due to smoking as a **means of comparison**. The age group of the study's patients was, on average, **61.5 years** - not really representative of a whole population, and the patients were **already in treatment for**

atherosclerosis. There is no information given on the lifestyle, smoking and/or eating habits of each patient. The study itself states:

"The study's weakness includes its observational nature, the lack of data on exercise, waist circumference and dietary intake of saturated fat and sources of cholesterol other than eggs, and the dependence on self-reporting of egg consumption and smoking history."

To then conclude:

*"Our findings suggest that regular consumption of egg yolk should be avoided by persons **at risk** of cardiovascular disease.* ***This hypothesis should be tested in a prospective study with more detailed information about diet, and other possible confounders such as exercise and waist circumference.***"

Oops, sounds to me like the study's findings are a bit cock-eyed! We don't know anything about the patients' lifestyle habits, we have no information on what was eaten with the egg yolks, we don't know if the egg whites were consumed at the same time, it is not clear if the people under study were smokers but the tone of the study leads to believe that at least some of them were, and there is no information on alcohol or sugar consumption. The study concludes that people at risk of cardiovascular disease should avoid egg yolks! The grammatical use of the conditional "should" in this case is interesting!

The media have certainly, in my opinion, singed their feathers on this one. They have once more taken a study that was done on a specific group of people, in specific conditions, with a specific health problem, and have attempted to fry the egg without any justification. What it boils down to is the use of sensational headlines in order to sell newspapers and the possibility of financial support from certain large companies who would still like us to believe that the problem is "fat" related and not "glucose" related. The media has egg on its face and it is time to eat crow!

One of the media articles concludes saying, *"Egg whites continue to be excellent!"* Although "using" a scientific study for the headline of the misconstrued article and its core message, the article's author did not see fit to cite any scientific study to back up the latter claim.

I have to say though that what shocks me about the study is that it repeats findings that came to light thirty or so years ago. There is no new evidence to support their findings. It is important to say that when they first studied cholesterol way back when, they were unaware that two types of cholesterol existed - one that is "bad" (LDL) and one that is "good" (HDL). The initial studies on the egg, all those years ago, showed that it contains a phenomenal amount of cholesterol - thus the previous scientists can be excused for their initial error, as they didn't have all the information to hand. As for the Canadian scientists today.... one wonders which came first, the scientist or the healthy egg nest?

Here are a few simple egg facts that I would like to share with you:

Yes, eggs contain a high amount of cholesterol - both LDL (the bad) and HDL (the good). The LDL cholesterol is mostly contained in the egg yolk, the HDL in the white. The consumption of the yolk and the white actually balances out the overall cholesterol levels, as there is more or less an equal amount of each type of cholesterol in each part of the egg. Magically, Nature knows how to do things - phew!

The egg always has been a valuable source of vitamins, minerals and protein - in fact there is a little health cocktail contained within its beautifully shaped shell, which contains high amounts of the major nutrients that our bodies require. But here's the hitch: the highest concentrate of these vitamins, minerals and oligo-elements are found in which part of the egg? Yes, the yolk! In an egg is found vitamin A, almost all of the vitamin B group, vitamin E, vitamin K, magnesium, calcium, phosphorus and potassium. It is jam-packed with iron and is a rare food-source of vitamin D. The protein content is similar to that of meat and is more easily assimilated by the human body. Eggs are also rich in omegas 3 and 6, necessary in the prevention of cardiovascular risks; oddly enough these omegas are contained in the yolk! Eating an egg without the yolk, just eating the white, has about the same nutritional value as eating cotton wool or baby-chick fluff.

The egg is classed in the group of Superfoods that absolutely should be included in our diets.

There is however, a difference that has to be taken into account, with regards to the type of eggs. Battery-hen laid eggs have higher amounts of LDL cholesterol and are practically devoid of any nutritional value. Wild-hen laid eggs are a perfect source of nourishment. Yes, I know that organic, wild-hen, free-range eggs are more expensive but let's face it, what we are looking for in food is the nutritional value. My philosophy is to buy better quality of which you don't eat perhaps quite so much - let's not forget that food is our first medicine.

It is also important to pay attention to the cooking methods. You will have noticed that overcooking an egg produces a greyish/green tinge around the yolk. This is due to the oxidation of the iron contained in the egg. The yolk requires a higher temperature than the white to solidify - a boiled egg with a runny yolk is then (supposedly!) easy to accomplish. Cooking over a certain temperature can also saturate the polyunsaturated fats contained in the egg along with the destruction of the liposoluble vitamins - so be careful with the cooking method and the temperature.

Eating starchy foods with eggs will cause the body to stockpile the fats found in the egg, which is not so good for the waistline. If you're still worried about the cholesterol levels, try omelettes with mushrooms/salmon/tuna - all delicious and all have a very good reputation of reducing LDL cholesterol levels. Accompany the lot with a delicious salad, chuck in some tomatoes for the colour and a little avocado, sprinkled with some nice vinaigrette made with olive-rapeseed-nut oil and you finish up with a fully balanced meal and I can assure you that you won't feel hungry for quite a few hours.

I think I may just have that for lunch!

To crack open the truth once and for all. It is not the consumption of foods containing cholesterol that is the problem. Studies, serious studies, done by independent non-government financed scientists, have shown that by reducing the glycemic load (sugar and starch) to an reasonable minimum is what reduces the levels of LDL cholesterol and triglycerides, and an increase in HDL cholesterol is notable, mostly because very naturally we will replace the high starch foods with more fibrous foods. The HDL cholesterol is good for our arteries and thus plays an important role in the prevention of cardiovascular disease.

The Power of the Pomegranate

The pomegranate, before the accidental discovery of antibiotics by Alexander Fleming, was used largely for its medicinal properties. It was used, particularly in Germany, as an antibiotic, an anti-viral and as a cure for influenza.

Recent scientific studies have attributed some rather extraordinary qualities to the pomegranate, the fruit and/or it's juice. One study has shown that the pomegranate is efficient in fighting not only against common flu but is also efficient against the famous and panic inducing H1N1 virus (swine flu), and H5N1 virus (bird flu), both of which have caused a fair amount of concern over recent years. Other studies have shown the pomegranate to be particularly useful against certain types of cancer – prostate, breast and lung cancer – in preventing the growth of tumours and aiding in the reduction of tumours. Pomegranate (juice) has also been shown to inactivate HIV, herpes, SARS and poxviruses and to render them non-infectious.

On a personal note: After a visit to family my 6-year old daughter came home one Sunday evening with a stinker of a cold, a bronchial cough, a high temperature and the beginnings of an ear infection. At this stage the family doctor would have certainly prescribed antibiotics but it was Sunday, no doctors were available. She had been prescribed "pneumorel", (by a family member who works in medicine), full of chemical ingredients designed to get the phlegm flowing. She had been taking this medicine for several days and all it was doing was making her throw up.

I immediately stopped the medicine, because it was making her throw up, and tapped into Nature's pharmacy. I gave her pomegranate juice, a third of a glass, three times a day. I told her that she should take it like medicine even if she didn't like the taste and the advantage would be that she wouldn't upset her tummy; the pomegranate is also very useful in regulating the intestinal flora. By the next day she was already coughing far less and her temperature had returned to normal. Within two days her lungs were much clearer and her ears had cleared. I made sure she blew her nose regularly to get rid of the bacteria filled gunk. Four days in, it was finished: no more cough; no more ear infection; no more temperature; and no more phlegm.

I'm not saying to stop the medicine prescribed by your own family doctor – I have no right to do so, but if you or your children are on medication for that kind of problem, adding in the pomegranate juice will, without doubt, be a help.

The Wonderful Wolfberry/Goji Berry

The best in Nature's pharmacy, the Goji berry is one of the most nutritiously dense fruits that exists on the planet and has been used in Chinese medicine for thousands of years in treating an array of health issues from the common cold to cancer.

It contains all eight amino acids, a large majority of trace minerals including calcium. It is the richest source of cartenoids of all known fruits on Earth and contains more beta-carotene than a carrot. Its antioxidant powers are 80 times more than even the pomegranate; it contains 500 times more vitamin C than an orange for an equivalent weight, and also contains some of the B group vitamins and vitamin E.

Studies have found these health inducing properties in Goji Berry:

- Goji boosts the immune system; that seems obvious. It improves eyesight and protects against cataracts and has been used in China for centuries to combat vision deficiencies.
- It protects the liver and prevents cellular destruction of the liver.
- It helps in reducing and relieving obesity through the calming of the pancreas and the levelling out of the blood sugars and the digestive metabolism. As such it is useful in the treatment of type II diabetes – again, the Goji has been used in a "dietary" optic for centuries in

Chinese medicine.

- It has been, and still is, used in the treatment of infertility, prolonging the cellular life, and preventing the destruction of sperm cells.

- It reduces hypertension and is used in the protection of cardiovascular health. As we get older the body's production of antioxidant enzymes that protect the cardiovascular system decreases; studies have shown that the consumption of Goji berry produces a 40% increase in the production of those enzymes, the antioxidants protecting the red blood cells from the action of oxygen radicals.

- It is used in the treatment of allergies as it reduces the antibodies associated with allergic reactions and is also useful in the treatment of psoriasis.

- It is used as an anti-inflammatory in the treatment of arthritis and inflammatory conditions.

- Interestingly the Goji berry induces the production of the same antioxidant enzyme that is useful in cardiovascular protection and prevents the free radicals from destroying it. This particular enzyme, superoxide dismutase, removes the free radicals that are greatly responsible for disease, and this removal results in beneficial outcomes for health.

- One of the most surprising and also miraculous properties of the Goji berry is its capacity to induce the production of interleukin-2. Interleukin-2 is the molecule that is used in chemotherapy; your body in fact knows how to make it itself and here's the very interesting part: self-produced interleukin-2 from within the body's own resources is far more efficient than the fabricated molecule that is used in the treatment of cancer, and without the unpleasant side effects of chemotherapy. Now, again, I am most certainly not saying to stop taking any cancer medication that you may be on and I'm definitely advising to check with your doctor and/or specialist before introducing Goji berry alongside any other type of cancer treatment. But the

Goji berry has shown to be efficient in reducing tumours for various different types of cancers including liver cancer and lung cancer and increases sensitivity during radiotherapy while enhancing the immune system. It is perhaps worth taking a look at with your Doctor and/or Specialist.

- On a lighter note, it's also an excellent aphrodisiac and very useful in the treatment of sexual impotence. An ancient Chinese proverb says:

> *"He who travels one thousand miles from home should not eat Goji"*

Apparently those particular qualities have been known for quite some time!

The only reservation that I have heard about concerning the Goji berry is its possible interaction with blood-thinning medication. The Goji naturally contains blood-thinning properties, so it could be a case of 'too much of a good thing!' If you are suffering from any kind of medical condition, it is always advised to consult your doctor or specialist before consuming Goji, or any other of the named Superfoods, alongside prescribed blood thinning treatments or any other medication that you may be taking.

The Stupendous Soursop

The Soursop is the most well-known, and well-hidden, cancer fighting treatment that exists on the planet – for cancers include lung, prostate, breast, liver, pancreatic, colon, etc. It has the advantage of killing only the cancerous cells while leaving the healthy cells intact, contrary to habitual chemotherapy and radiotherapy treatments. It also reduces the side effects of chemotherapy and radiotherapy, whilst boosting the immune system. It helps to improve digestive health and also increases the blood and platelet count.

Other properties of the Soursop fruit are: migraine relief; anaemia prevention; treatment of liver disorders; improvement of bone health through a better assimilation of calcium; anti-inflammatory properties; pain relief in conditions such as arthritis and rheumatism; and increased energy levels. The leaves, roots, bark and sap of the Soursop tree have also been shown to be efficient in the treatment of: skin disorders such as eczema; coughs and fevers; dysentery and; oddly enough, in the treatment of head lice. Teas made from the leaves have also shown to prevent the over-production of insulin, protect the pancreas and level out the blood sugar levels.

There is another tiny herb that should be mentioned in conjunction with Soursop, as it has many of the same qualities, specifically as a potent cancer-fighting agent, which is Saffron. As a spice, it is extremely costly but is extremely powerful in very small doses.

However, and there is a however, some studies have shown that an overconsumption of Soursop may prove to be somewhat toxic, causing some digestive problems. Pregnant women should also be cautious as, while the fruit contains high amounts of folic acid, which is necessary for the growth of the embryo and the foetus, too high an intake of Soursop fruit may also cause uterine contractions, which could ultimately lead to miscarriage. The antibacterial properties may also have an adverse effect on the digestive system with too high a consumption of the fruit, destroying the intestinal flora and causing diarrhoea. There doesn't seem to be much evidence of those last claims, there are no specific studies, but I believe it is always best to be on the safe side. Consult your doctor if you have the slightest doubt.

Here is a short list of just some of the other Superfoods that we can find easily in our own kitchens and their benefits:

All the Little Oily Fishes

The scientific community were baffled, for quite some time, by the dietary habits of the Inuit people who ate a lot of oily fish but very little vegetables and absolutely no carbohydrates, as vegetables were in rare supply and carbohydrates were practically non-existent. The scientists could not understand how these people could eat so much 'fat' and have such low rates of cardiovascular disease. As it turns out, oily fish are a rich source of omegas, essential in the prevention of arterial and coronary problems.

They are a rich source of minerals. Sardines contain vitamin D and natural calcium that is well assimilated by the human body, as long as you eat the fish-bones along with flesh.

The omegas in the oily fish have also been suggested to be extremely beneficial in relieving depression, anxiety disorders and nervous agitation and can combat the inflammation connected to arthritis and rheumatism.

Again, whether it's true or not, it doesn't really matter – eating oily fish is not going to do you any harm and if it can do you some good then so much the better!

Of course, there is a lot of concern these days about eating fish due to the conditions of our oceans. The high levels of pollution, toxic dumping, oil excavation, oil spills, off-coast fracking, and nuclear accidents have rendered our oceans unsafe and, of course, all of that enters into the food chain. For the seas to overcome the high levels of pollution, that they have been subjected to over the last fifty or so years, could require anything up to 10,000 years.

Fish farming, like battery hens, that keep the fish confined in waters that can stagnate (though certain fish farms in bonnie Scotland and Norway have their cages at sea, so the water doesn't stagnate), to where the fish are fed a diet that is not naturally their own and where they are pumped full of antibiotics to "protect" them from diseases due to the water conditions, is not a much better solution.

I have to admit that I tend to hesitate when buying fish for all of the above reasons - the "new" and more expensive "organic" fish does not seem a huge improvement. These are still fish that are farmed, just minus the antibiotics and the pesticides in the feed. And it seems very odd that wild fish are not allowed to carry the label "organic" when they are, in fact, the most natural source of organic fish and often inhabit areas where the waters would be cleaner than elsewhere.

So, where possible take a swim on the wild side!

Gobble Some Turkey

It's one of the leanest sources of meat on the planet, which probably explains why it's so dry and has a taste similar to that of cardboard – that's just my opinion! I get round that by marinating it which makes it that little bit more juicy. The proteins are excellent and very well assimilated by us humans but, more interestingly, turkey is a rich source of minerals that we don't find in all foods – selenium and zinc for example – and B group vitamins, which are useful in heart disease and cancer prevention.

Amazing Avocado

Avocado contains mono-unsaturated fat, magnesium, potassium, vitamin E, folic acid and can help in the regulation of blood pressure; prevention of migraines; prevention of type II diabetes; decrease of LDL cholesterol; and an increase of HDL cholesterol. It is effective in aiding the assimilation of nutrients from other food sources and useful for women in regulating the hormones oestrogen and progesterone.

But, gentlemen do not feel left out! Recent studies have shown that the nutrients in avocado are an effective aid in the combat against prostate cancer.

And they taste so good! *Try them with a garlic vinaigrette (half a teaspoon of mustard, 3 tsp of cider vinegar, 9 tsp of olive oil, a dash of balsamic vinegar, 1 crushed clove of garlic or more to taste, salt and pepper), cut the avocadoes in half, scoop them out of their skin, spoon in some vinaigrette...* What more could we ask for?

Any Green Will Do!

Broccoli, Cabbage, Sprouts, Spinach, Kale, etc, etc.
These greens are full of iron, vitamins, nutrients, zinc, potassium and calcium – all Nature-made and all absorbable by the human being. They are all an incredible source of fibre, are useful in the prevention of many diseases such as: type II diabetes; high blood pressure; cardiovascular illnesses; cancer; cataracts; birth defects such as spina bifida; osteoporosis; and help in blood clotting. They also boost the immune system – mix them with some garlic and you have a rather powerful little anti-viral cocktail.
Well, I think that just about covers all our needs!

For best results with broccoli, I either eat them raw with a little bit of salt or lightly steam them. If they are overcooked, they lose their colour, take on a rather bitter taste and lose a lot of their goodness through the cooking process.

Many people eat spinach cooked, but it's said that when it is cooked it becomes quite toxic? I've surprised many of my friends by serving it to them raw in salads, young leaves are best – it has an amazing peppery taste and makes for a nice array of shades of green and flavours if mixed with other salad leaves.

Cabbage and sprouts: I tend to cook them so that they stay crisp and still have some bite to them but rarely eat them raw. I personally find the raw taste too pungent but when they're overcooked they become rather bitter and also lose their goodness.

The Magic Mushroom

No, I don't mean the hallucinogenic kind, just the ordinary kind will do but, of course, that's your own personal choice!

Amongst many of its other powerful attributes, mushrooms, like sardines, are a combined source of edible vitamin D and calcium! They contain a very high concentration of vitamins and minerals that help the body to prevent, you guessed it already: heart disease; cancer; high blood pressure; and type II diabetes. But the powerful little mushroom doesn't just stop there. No, no, no, it also lowers LDL cholesterol levels; increases HDL cholesterol levels; regulates blood sugar; protects the body from free radicals; boosts the immune system and is very useful in the treatment of ulcers and ulcerous wounds. And if that wasn't enough already, it also, although it is a fungus, helps and prevents against bacterial and fungal infections.

Terrific Tomatoes

A power ball of vital nutrients, which includes a special little molecule called lycopene. In France, the onion is described as the vegetable of longevity, but the tomato will get you to a ripe old age in fine form. Lycopene is a powerful antioxidant and interestingly, can also protect your skin from the damaging rays of the sun – literally protecting you from the inside out. The tomato is also full of carotene, polyphenols, most of the vitamin B group, vitamin E, folic acid, potassium, manganese, magnesium and zinc. Hence we have all the usual advantages – protection against cancer, high blood pressure, heart disease and type II diabetes.

Just as an aside, a little anecdote about my daughter Colleen, for all those who say that children don't like vegetables:
One day, when she was about 15 months old and had just started to walk, I had left a huge bowl of tomato, cucumber and garlic salad in the kitchen. I went off to do something else and when I came back the bowl had gone! Then I quickly realized that she had taken the bowl, climbed into her high chair and eaten the lot in the short time that I'd left the room! Though she'd eaten everybody's lunch, how do you tell your child off for eating vegetables?

Children don't like *all* vegetables – true and the trick, which I'm sure you know already, is to find the ones that they like to eat. It might not be terribly varied but we all know the importance of veg in our diets, whether for adults in order to maintain our infrastructure or children for developing it.

Great Garlic!

Powerful antibiotic and a powerful booster for the immune system, perhaps because the odour will keep those other people and their infectious germs at a safe distance!
But the little garlic bulb won't just protect you from vampires; it will also protect your heart, your arteries and your eyes. It's an aid against cerebral aging, immune disorders, cancer, and is not only a powerful antioxidant but is also a powerful anti-inflammatory.

Beans and Lentils

Full of iron and vitamins, they are also a very interesting source of protein that is well assimilated when the beans or lentils are eaten with some kind of whole cereal. They assist in reducing LDL cholesterol levels, hypertension, cardiovascular protection, combat obesity through the levelling out of blood sugars, and also contain cancer-fighting agents.

Most beans, apart from lentils, split peas and barley, require overnight soaking and a long cooking time. An option is to use tinned beans, however there is some question as to whether the Bisphenol A that is used in the lining of tin cans presents a dangerous level of toxicity. Again, the fact that there is question around that tends to lead to the conclusion that if in doubt, it's best to avoid. On a more practical and happier note, cooked beans freeze very well, so that can be another option.

You can add to this list the most notable among the commonly found Superfoods:
Buckwheat, Oats, Nuts, Almonds, Walnuts, Dark Chocolate (70% cocoa minimum), raw cocoa, flax seeds, honey, blueberries, cranberries, all herbs, cinnamon, olive oil, red wine and... champagne! Now, if that weren't reason enough to celebrate!

"I'd like the mushroom and tuna omelette with a spinach, tomato and avocado salad, served with a garlic vinaigrette dressing, followed by the lentil and turkey stuffed cabbage leaves. For dessert, I'd like the dark chocolate mousse sprinkled with walnuts and almonds and I'll accompany all that with a nice glass of champagne!"

Would you care to join me?

Final Words

Nature has provided for us, since the beginning of time, with everything we need to be healthy and to live well. We have a full Natural pharmacy at our disposal; we can grow that pharmacy in our own gardens.

Nature has also doted us with a marvellous human capacity to understand our surroundings, to navigate through our surroundings and to love our surroundings.

It is up to us, as thinking, conscious beings, to respect, take care of and to wisely use this miraculous gift that is part of us and that we are a part of.

> *"A human being is a part of a whole, called by us _universe_, a part limited in time and space. He experiences himself, his thoughts and feelings as something separated from the rest... a kind of optical delusion of his consciousness. This delusion is a kind of prison for us, restricting us to our personal desires and to affection for a few persons nearest to us. Our task must be to free ourselves from this prison by widening our circle of compassion to embrace all living creatures and the whole of nature in its beauty." – Albert Einstein*

Namaste,
Love and Light,
Rachel

Resources:

- Some Inspiring Books on Food:

Michel Montignac, Eat Yourself Slim
Thierry Souccar, Santé, Mensonges et Propagande
Dr. Peter J. D'Adamo, Eat Right for Your Type
Dr. Alain Delabos, Chrononutrition (book in French)
Dr. John Yudkin, Pure, White and Deadly

- Some Inspiring Books on the Nature of the Human Experience:

Sydney Banks, The Enlightened Gardener
Sydney Banks, The Missing Link
Michael Neill, The Inside Out Revolution
Jack Pransky, Somebody Should Have Told Us
Elsie Spittle, Our True Identity
Jamie Smart, Clarity

- Some Audiovisual Resources on Food:

Dr. Robert Lustig, Sugar The Bitter Truth
Dr. Robert Lustig, The Skinny on Obesity
Morgan Spurlock, Supersize Me
BBC Documentary, The Men Who Made Us Fat

- Some AudioVisual Resources on the Human Experience:

Tikun, Innate Health Conferences:

http://www.tikun.co.uk/events/spiritual-wellbeing-events/2011-innate-health-conference-844.php

http://www.tikun.co.uk/missinglink/2012videos.php

Three Principles Movies:

http://www.threeprinciplesmovies.com/

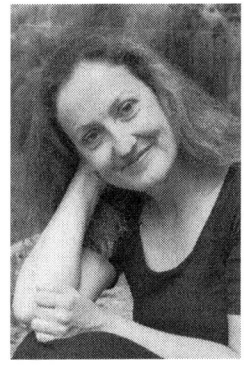

Rachel Norwood is a Three Principles Practitioner and author of "The Gentle Path to Definitive Weight Loss" and the forthcoming book "The Gentle Path to Fulfilment", the French version, "Le Chemin Doux vers l'Epanouissement."

She works with individuals and groups, both in English and French, helping them understand their relationship to their thoughts and how their thinking shapes their reality and perception. She aids her clients in a variety of areas; weight loss, relationships, personal accomplishment, overcoming stress and performance anxiety, creativity, and accompanies them in a life-changing experience that does not require techniques or hard work, nor motivation and willpower but rather in assisting her clients in accessing their own Wisdom, Resilience and Innate Well Being.

Rachel has been practicing and working with the Three Principles specifically for over a year with extraordinary results both for herself and for her clients. She first came across the Principles and the Inside-Out understanding of the human experience on joining Michael Neill's "Living from the Inside-Out" program. Recognizing the power of this understanding, she pursued her learning with Michael Neill's "Coaching from the Inside-Out" program, and the recent 2013 "Living from the Inside-Out" programs, deepening her knowledge further through the teachings at Tikun London (Innate health Conferences of 2011 and 2012) and with the recorded and written teachings of Sydney Banks, the founder of this new approach in psychology, along with materials provided by other eminent Practitioners in the field.

Printed in Great Britain
by Amazon

41567591R00115